Miscellaneous Considerations in Inflammatory Bowel Disease

Edited by Vinaya Gaduputi

Published in London, United Kingdom

Miscellaneous Considerations in Inflammatory Bowel Disease
http://dx.doi.org/10.5772/intechopen.1000411
Edited by Vinaya Gaduputi

Contributors
Ahmad Kasem, Anam Fahad, Anna Buczynska, Asfand Yar Cheema, Aychin I. Hasanova, Bahadir Kartal, Emin Kh. Verdiyev, Ferid V. Guliyev, Giuseppe Leoncini, Gulustan H. Babayeva, Gunay V. Asadova, Habil M. Huseynov, Hammad Qureshi, Hikmet I. Ibrahimli, Hira Tahir, Jamal S. Musayev, Katalin E. Müller, Mishaal Munir, Muhammad Ali Khan, Rachele Del Sordo, Rahimeen Rajpar, Rashad A. Hasanov, Sabina Wiecek, Sarayu Bhogoju, Sergiy V. Holub, Simona Ronchetti, Somia Jamal Sheikh, Syed Adeel Hassan, Tunzala A. Maharramova, Umud R. Mahmudov, Vinaya Gaduputi, Vincenzo Villanacci

First published in London, United Kingdom, 2024 by IntechOpen
IntechOpen is the global imprint of INTECHOPEN LIMITED, registered in England and Wales, registration number: 11086078, 167-169 Great Portland Street, London, W1W 5PF, United Kingdom

British Library Cataloguing-in-Publication Data
A catalogue record for this book is available from the British Library

Additional hard and PDF copies can be obtained from orders@intechopen.com

Miscellaneous Considerations in Inflammatory Bowel Disease
Edited by Vinaya Gaduputi
p. cm.
Print ISBN 978-1-83769-691-8
Online ISBN 978-1-83769-690-1
eBook (PDF) ISBN 978-1-83769-692-5

For EU product safety concerns:
IN TECH d.o.o., Prolaz Marije Krucifikse Kozulić 3, 51000 Rijeka, Croatia,
info@intechopen.com or visit our website at intechopen.com.

Meet the editor

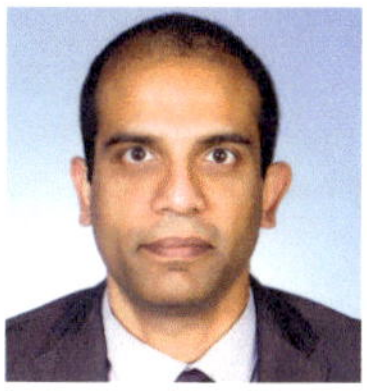

Dr. Vinaya Gaduputi is an Attending Physician at Blanchard Valley Health System, OH, USA. He is the author and co-author of more than 100 papers published in well-indexed journals and more than 130 abstracts accepted at major international gastroenterology conferences. He has thousands of citations by researchers in the field of gastroenterology. He is the recipient of several awards, including the Presidential Poster Award by the American College of Gastroenterology and the Poster of Distinction Award by Digestive Disease Week. Dr. Gaduputi previously served as Director of the Division of Gastroenterology and Hepatology at SBH Health System, NY, USA. He also served as Assistant Program Director, Internal Medicine Residency at SBH Health System, and Assistant Program Director, Gastroenterology Fellowship Program, Brooklyn Medical Center, NY.

Contents

Preface

Inflammatory Bowel Disease (IBD) is a complex and multifaceted condition that affects millions of people worldwide. The burden of IBD is growing, with increasing incidence and prevalence globally. This book provides a comprehensive overview of the unique and important aspects of IBD, with a focus on practical, evidence-based information that can be applied in clinical practice.

The landscape of IBD treatment has changed dramatically over the past few decades. Advances in medical technology, combined with a deeper understanding of the disease's pathophysiology, have led to the development of novel therapeutic strategies. These include the use of biologics, small molecules, and personalized medicine approaches, which have significantly improved the prognosis for many patients with IBD. Despite these advances, many challenges remain. The etiology of IBD is still not fully understood, and there is a need for better predictive models to guide treatment decisions. Furthermore, the management of IBD is complicated by the disease's heterogeneous nature, with patients often presenting with a wide range of symptoms and disease severities.

This book delves into various aspects of IBD, from its pathophysiology and clinical presentation to the latest advances in diagnostic techniques and treatment strategies. Dedicated sections discuss often-overlooked but equally important considerations.

The book opens with an introductory chapter.

Chapter 2 provides a comprehensive overview of the unique challenges and considerations related to body composition in pediatric patients with IBD. Children with IBD often experience growth delays and alterations in body composition, which can have significant implications for their overall health and disease management. This chapter delves into the factors influencing these changes, the methods for assessing body composition in this population, and the potential strategies for addressing these issues. It is our hope that this chapter will serve as a valuable resource for clinicians and researchers working in the field of pediatric IBD.

In Chapter 3, we explore two common gastrointestinal issues that can complicate the clinical picture of pediatric IBD: lactose intolerance and small intestinal bacterial overgrowth (SIBO). Both conditions can mimic or exacerbate IBD symptoms, making diagnosis and management challenging. This chapter provides a comprehensive understanding of these conditions in the context of pediatric IBD, discussing their pathophysiology, clinical presentation, diagnostic methods, and management strategies. By shedding light on these often-overlooked aspects of pediatric IBD, we hope to equip clinicians with the knowledge needed to provide holistic care to their young patients.

Chapter 4 provides an overview of the evolution of diagnostic pathways in IBD. It begins with a review of traditional diagnostic methods, discussing their strengths and limitations. The chapter then transitions into an exploration of newer diagnostic approaches, including advancements in imaging, endoscopy, and biomarker discovery. The aim is to highlight how these new pathways have improved our ability to diagnose IBD accurately and promptly, thereby enabling more effective management of the disease. This chapter serves as a valuable resource for clinicians and researchers seeking to understand the past, present, and future of IBD diagnosis.

Therapeutic drug monitoring forms the basis of Chapter 5. As the treatment landscape for IBD continues to evolve, it is essential for clinicians to understand how to monitor drug levels and adjust treatment plans accordingly to optimize patient outcomes. With the advent of new drug therapies, understanding the pharmacokinetics and pharmacodynamics of these medications has become increasingly important. This chapter discusses the principles of therapeutic drug monitoring, its application in optimizing drug therapy for IBD, and the latest advancements in this field.

Chapter 6 discusses the critical area of identifying predictors of nonresponse to ongoing conservative therapy IBD. Understanding these predictors is crucial in the management of IBD, as it can guide clinicians in tailoring treatment plans and potentially prevent unnecessary disease progression and complications. The chapter provides a comprehensive overview of the current knowledge on this topic, discussing various clinical, genetic, and pharmacological predictors, and how they can be used to inform treatment decisions.

Finally, we delve into surgical interventions in IBD. While the goal is always to manage IBD with medical therapy, surgery is sometimes necessary. The final chapter discusses the various surgical options, their indications, and potential complications. It also explores the decision-making process that leads to surgery, including when and how to make this difficult decision.

This textbook is a valuable resource for clinicians, researchers, and students alike. It is our hope that it will contribute to improving the care and quality of life for patients with IBD.

This textbook is the result of the collective efforts of numerous experts in the field of gastroenterology, each bringing their unique perspectives and expertise to the table. Leading this endeavor is the Chief Editor, Dr. Vinaya Gaduputi, a gastroenterologist and a hepatologist. Dr. Gaduputi is currently affiliated with the Division of Gastroenterology & Hepatology, Department of Internal Medicine, Blanchard Valley Hospital System, USA.

We would like to express our gratitude to all the authors for their invaluable contributions and to the patients and their families, who teach us so much about resilience and hope. We hope that this textbook will serve as a comprehensive guide to IBD, providing you with the knowledge and insights needed to better understand and manage this complex condition. We are grateful for your interest in our work and hope that you find this resource valuable in your journey to understand and manage IBD. Thank you for choosing this textbook as your guide in the fascinating and ever-evolving world of inflammatory bowel disease.

Vinaya Gaduputi MD FACG
Blanchard Valley Health System,
Findlay, OH, USA

Chapter 1

Introductory Chapter: Miscellaneous Considerations in Inflammatory Bowel Disease

Vinaya Gaduputi

1. Introduction

Inflammatory Bowel Disease (IBD) stands as a formidable challenge in the landscape of gastroenterological disorders, encompassing two primary entities—Crohn's disease (CD) and ulcerative colitis (UC). Characterized by chronic inflammation of the gastrointestinal tract, IBD's impact extends far beyond the confines of the digestive system, affecting the lives of millions worldwide. With an increasing global prevalence, the burden of IBD has evolved into a complex interplay of genetic predispositions, environmental factors, and immune dysregulation.

The incidence of IBD has witnessed a notable surge over recent decades, imposing a significant societal and economic burden. According to the Global Burden of Disease database, IBD affected approximately 4.9 million people globally in 2019 [1], with a projected increase in the years to come. The toll on the quality of life for those afflicted is profound, as the disease often strikes during the prime years of adulthood, interrupting careers, education, and personal relationships. Furthermore, the economic burden stemming from healthcare costs and lost productivity places IBD at the forefront of public health concerns.

As our understanding of IBD deepens, so too does our recognition of the multifaceted challenges it presents. From a clinical perspective, IBD manifests with a spectrum of symptoms, including abdominal pain, diarrhea, weight loss, and fatigue. However, the heterogeneity of the disease poses a significant diagnostic and therapeutic challenge. The intricate interplay of genetic, environmental, and immunological factors contributes to the varied clinical presentations observed among individuals with IBD. Moreover, the elusive etiology of IBD remains a central enigma. While genetic susceptibility is acknowledged, environmental triggers, such as diet, microbiome composition, and lifestyle, play pivotal roles in disease onset and progression. The intricate crosstalk between the gut microbiota and the host immune system has emerged as a key player in the pathogenesis of IBD, adding layers of complexity to our understanding of the disease [2].

Understanding IBD necessitates a journey through its historical trajectory. IBD was first recognized as early as late eighteenth century [3]. The distinct entities of CD and UC were gradually delineated as unique clinical entities with diverse presentations and pathological characteristics in the twentieth century [4]. Over the ensuing decades, strides in diagnostic imaging, endoscopy, and molecular biology have enriched our comprehension of IBD. The advent of genetic studies has unearthed a multitude of susceptibility genes, shedding light on the hereditary aspects of the disease.

There is a need to embark on an exploration of newer challenges in IBD while delving into specific facets of IBD, providing a nuanced understanding of the disease and equipping healthcare professionals, researchers, and students with the knowledge needed to navigate the complexities of IBD diagnosis and management.

2. Evolution of IBD management: navigating the shifting landscape

The diagnostic journey in IBD has undergone a transformative evolution, shaped by advances in technology, molecular understanding, and diagnostic modalities. One needs to explore the dynamic landscape of diagnostic pathways for IBD, meticulously examining the historical perspectives alongside contemporary approaches. From traditional clinical assessments to cutting-edge biomarkers and imaging technologies, the diagnostic armamentarium has exponentially increased. As we traverse the terrain of old and new diagnostic paths, one has to acknowledge the pivotal roles of endoscopy, serological markers, genetic testing, and emerging technologies, offering a comprehensive exploration of the multifaceted strategies employed in the accurate identification and classification of Inflammatory Bowel Diseases.

In recent years, the therapeutic arsenal against IBD has expanded, reflecting a paradigm shift in our approach to disease management. Traditional treatment modalities, including aminosalicylates, corticosteroids, and immunomodulators, remain integral components of IBD care. However, the emergence of biologic agents has revolutionized the treatment landscape, providing targeted interventions that interrupt specific pathways in the inflammatory cascade. Furthermore, the advent of small molecule inhibitors has added another dimension to IBD therapeutics. These oral agents target intracellular signaling pathways, offering an alternative for patients who may not respond to or tolerate biologic therapies. The era of personalized medicine is dawning upon IBD, with a growing emphasis on tailoring treatment strategies based on individual patient profiles, disease phenotypes, and biomarker profiles.

There is a need to have a structured approach to navigate through the intricate landscape of predictors influencing non-response to ongoing conservative therapy in patients with IBD. Unraveling the factors contributing to treatment resistance, equips healthcare professionals with a deeper understanding of the complexities surrounding IBD management, paving the way for more personalized and efficacious interventions.

A very important subset of patients with IBD is the pediatric age group comprising up to 10% of all the cases [5]. In the realm of pediatric gastroenterology, the burden of Inflammatory Bowel Disease (IBD) presents a unique set of challenges that necessitate a nuanced understanding of its multifaceted nature. Physicians must be cognizant of the pediatric aspect of IBD and of the intricate interplay between the disease burden and specific considerations such as body composition. Beyond the conventional focus on symptoms and inflammation, one has to consider the impact of IBD on the developing body, emphasizing the critical role of body composition in pediatric patients. Additionally, there are issues such as the coexistence of Lactose Intolerance and Small Intestinal Bacterial Overgrowth (SIBO), adding layers to the diagnostic and therapeutic considerations.

There is a pivotal evolving role of surgical interventions in the context of IBD. As a multifaceted and dynamic field, the role of surgery in managing IBD has witnessed significant advancements over the years. One needs to have a comprehensive overview of the surgical approaches employed in the treatment of IBD, encompassing

DOI: http://dx.doi.org/10.5772/intechopen.1004396

both Crohn's disease and ulcerative colitis. Drawing on a wealth of scholarly research that deals with surgical interventions in achieving sustained remission and improving the overall quality of life for patients with IBD and through a critical analysis of these studies, physicians should seek to elucidate the nuanced relationship between surgery and IBD management.

Through an evidence-based exploration, we have strived to enhance the comprehension of healthcare professionals. By integrating relevant research findings and clinical insights, we hope to provide an indispensable resource for clinicians navigating the complexities of Inflammatory Bowel Disease management.

Author details

Vinaya Gaduputi
Blanchard Valley Health System, OH, USA

*Address all correspondence to: vgaduputi@bvhealthsystem.org

References

[1] Wang R, Li Z, Liu S, Zhang D. Global, regional and national burden of inflammatory bowel disease in 204 countries and territories from 1990 to 2019: A systematic analysis based on the Global Burden of Disease Study 2019. BMJ Open. 2023;**13**(3):e065186

[2] Quaglio AEV, Grillo TG, De Oliveira ECS, Di Stasi LC, Sassaki LY. Gut microbiota, inflammatory bowel disease and colorectal cancer. World Journal of Gastroenterology. 2022;**28**(30):4053-4060

[3] Actis GC, Pellicano R, Fagoonee S, Ribaldone DG. History of inflammatory bowel diseases. Journal of Clinical Medicine. 2019;**8**(11):1970

[4] Kirsner JB. Historical origins of current IBD concepts. World Journal of Gastroenterology. 2001;**7**(2):175-184

[5] Bouhuys M, Lexmond WS, van Rheenen PF. Pediatric inflammatory bowel disease. Pediatrics. 2023;**151**(1):e2022058037

Chapter 2

Body Composition in Pediatric Inflammatory Bowel Disease

Katalin E. Müller

Abstract

Malnutrition and assessment of body composition is an important topic in inflammatory bowel disease. The pathomechanism of malnutrition is complex and related to anorexia, abnormal digestion, malabsorption, and chronic inflammation. Anthropometric parameters and BMI are not precise to reflect the nutritional status. Meanwhile, recent studies emphasize that low fat-free mass, especially, sarcopenia is associated with a worse prognosis, such as an increased risk for surgery, biological therapy, and disease complications. On the other hand, obesity and increased fat mass are also associated with poor outcomes in patients with inflammatory bowel disease. Furthermore, the dosage of some drugs may need adjustment in the case of obese patients with inflammatory bowel disease.

Keywords: body composition, sarcopenia, inflammatory bowel disease, fat-free mass, malnutrition

1. Introduction

Malnutrition has always been the focus of inflammatory bowel disease [IBD] management. Nowadays, it has gained even more attention as we learned more about body composition. Malnutrition and impaired body composition are significantly contributed to unmeasured morbidity in IBD. Altered body composition may influence the course of the illness, response to therapies, outcomes of surgery, and quality of life [QoL].

However, the practice of calculating body mass index [BMI] may fail, since a deficit of lean mass can be masked by fat mass [FM]. Advanced techniques should be used to discover the alteration of body composition. Body composition analysis divides the body into compartments of lean mass and fat mass.

Multiple factors are responsible for the alteration of body composition. Chronic inflammatory activity modifies nutrient utilization, malabsorption, decreased appetite, and physical activity also contribute to the loss of the metabolically active fat-free mass [FFM]. IBD is associated with impaired body composition including reduced bone density and skeletal muscle mass. Furthermore, as obesity becomes widespread, the role of adipose tissue in the inflammatory process has been recognized also in patients with IBD.

Clinical awareness of body composition and appropriate management are a highlight to improve disease outcomes and QoL of patients with IBD.

2. Malnutrition in inflammatory bowel disease

Malnutrition can be defined as "a state resulting from lack of intake or uptake of nutrition that leads to altered body composition (decreased FFM) and body cell mass leading to diminished physical and mental function and impaired clinical outcome from disease" [1]. Malnutrition is related with poor prognosis, impaired body composition, physical and emotional well-being, QoL, and body form. Altered body composition, such as loss of FFM or skeletal muscle mass (SMM), has been demonstrated even in the case of normal BMI.

The IBD itself and its treatment (e.g. systemic corticosteroids) influence the nutritional status and body composition through several mechanisms. First, reduced appetite, nausea, and abdominal pain result in reduced energy and nutrient intake. Micronutrient and vitamin deficiencies along with inflammatory cytokines can impair taste sensation that can contribute to anorexia. Second, diarrhea and malabsorption contribute to the loss of nutrients due to impaired epithelial integrity, bacterial overgrowth, and reduction of absorptive surfaces (intestinal resection, enteric fistulas). Third, inflammatory cytokines (IL-1, TNF- α, IL-6) alter energy metabolism, protein turnover, and increase energy requirements, thus they exert an effect on body composition and trigger signs of cachexia, such as anorexia, and loss of skeletal muscle mass [2]. In addition, patients with chronic gastrointestinal symptoms often start restrictive diets that may increase the risk of malnutrition [3]. Finally, low physical activity due to fatigue and active symptoms can also impact body composition. Regarding the medications, it is well-known, that glucocorticoid therapy is associated with an increase in FM and has catabolic effect on lean mass, meanwhile anti-TNF seems to be effective also in the improvement of FFM. Additionally, anorexigenic side effects of some medications may also complicate the problem of undernutrition in IBD (**Figure 1**) [4].

Body composition includes also fat compartments that can be divided into subcutaneous and visceral fat. Mesenteric adipose tissue belonging to visceral fat has an important role in the regulation of inflammatory processes due to the production of several pro-inflammatory cytokines and mediators. Adipose tissue

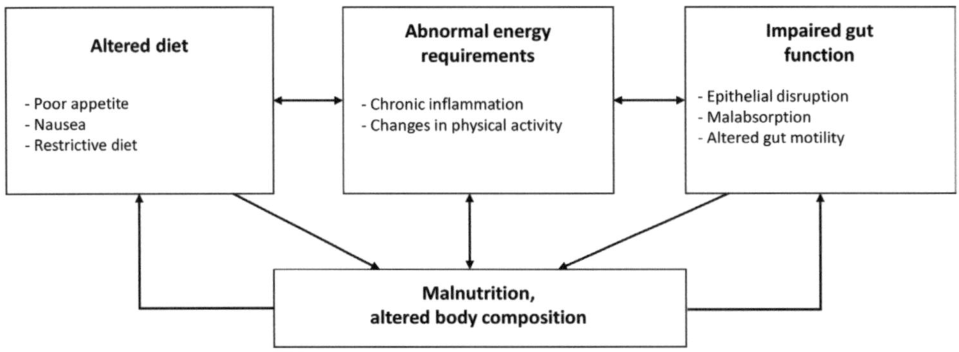

Figure 1.
Pathophysiological factors leading to impaired body composition in patients with inflammatory bowel disease.

due to its pro-inflammatory nature and loss of SMM are both associated with poor outcomes in IBD independently from each other. Meanwhile, skeletal muscle releasing anti-inflammatory cytokines (myokines, IL-15) may be protective against poor outcomes [5].

3. Body composition and its measurement

Earlier, BMI was essential in the assessment of nutritional status, however, evidence suggests, that BMI is not precise enough. Although BMI is a useful anthropometric parameter, it is not able to discriminate between excess body fat and increased lean mass [6]. Some studies in IBD patients highlighted that alteration in body parameters, mostly reduced lean mass, despite normal BMI [7].

In everyday practice to evaluate body composition the two-component model is still the most widely used model of body composition (**Figure 2**). The two-component model differentiates the body into FM (which consists of the visceral and subcutaneous adipose tissue), and FFM, (active metabolizer part of the body). FFM consists of the total body water (including intra- and extracellular water), total body mineral (mainly bone tissue) and protein, and essential lipids (involved in cellular physiology, e.g. phospholipids). Lean body mass (LBM) is frequently used as a synonym for FFM. However, theoretically lean body mass is composed of total body water and mineral, proteins, but not essential lipid components [8]. The weight of essential lipids is negligible, and FFM and LM are applicable to characterize the metabolically active part of the body. A third important compartment is skeletal muscle mass (SMM) included in FFM and LBM, which is also an essential parameter to characterize body composition and sarcopenia in IBD. In contrast to the two-component model, multicomponent models minimize the assumptions, rather they measure each component separately [9]. The three-component model divides body weight into fat-free dry tissue, fat, water. The four-component model separates fat-free dry tissue into protein and mineral [9].

LBM has several functions, and LBM deficits are associated with morbidity via loss of muscle mass and strength, and altered metabolism. In addition, LBM has an important role in the regulation of bone mass, by applying stress to bones,

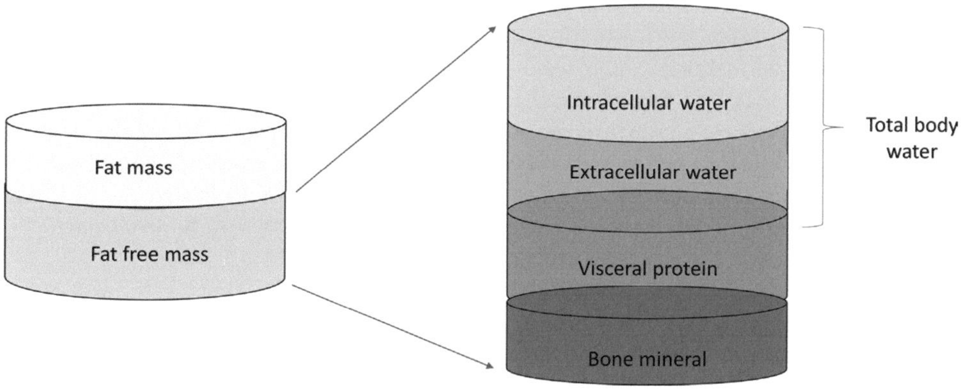

Figure 2.
Two-component model of body composition.

additionally. In contrast, an increase in fat mass is associated with elevated inflammatory markers [10].

3.1 Regulation of body composition compartments

Body composition is influenced by several factors like geography, ethnicity, age, sex. Furthermore, body composition compartments are in interaction with each other throughout hormonal regulation and cell-signaling networks [11]. Pathological conditions can modulate the balance leading to altered body composition.

Adipose tissue takes part in the regulation of metabolism, but is also known to produce pro-inflammatory cytokines. Mesenterial visceral fat ("creeping fat") has a special role in IBD, especially in CD. Visceral fat releases adipokines (leptin and resistin) and pro-inflammatory cytokines (TNF-α, IFN-γ, IL-6, IL-1). Bacterial lipopolysaccharides induce resistin production, which promotes the secretion of TNF-α and IL-12, activates mononuclear cells, and interact with bone mass, as well. Leptin induces mononuclear and CD4+ T cells and promotes the development of Th1 response.

As mentioned above bone mass is influenced by resistin, which increases the number of osteoclasts, leading to loss of bone mass. Adiponectin also exerts a negative effect on bone mass. In addition, it is well-documented that the bone mass is also affected by chronic inflammation that alters the balance between osteoblasts and osteoclasts via TNF-α, IL-1, and IL-6 [11].

As an important component of FFM, the SMM takes part in the metabolism of glucose and protein metabolism. Furthermore, SMM and physical activity can increase bone mineral density and induce the production of anti-inflammatory cytokines and myokines [12]. In chronic inflammation, the elevated TNF-α and IL-6 induce protein degradation and reduction of myofibrillar proteins via growth hormone resistance in the liver and muscles.

3.2 Assessment of body composition

Anthropometrical parameters such as weight, height, BMI, and body circumferences are essential to assess nutritional status and body composition. However, in clinical practice, impaired body composition often remains unrecognized if only BMI is used. A few studies have demonstrated that BMI is not sensitive to detect a low lean mass, especially since it does not indicate sarcopenia in the case of co-existing obesity (sarcopenic obesity) [4, 13]. The detailed characterization of body composition compartments is only feasible with special techniques. Numerous non-invasive techniques are available to assess body composition for clinical and research purposes. Certainly, all of them have their advantages and disadvantages.

Skinfold thickness measurement is an easy and inexpensive method for assessing fat mass in clinical practice, however, the ratio of subcutaneous and total body fat remains uncertain. **Dual-energy x-ray absorptiometry (DEXA)** is also a widespread and at the same time reliable tool to estimate lean and fat mass, and bone density. Though, it is expensive and works with radiation exposure [14].

Bioelectrical impedance analysis (BIA) is another non-invasive, safe, easy-to-use method, that can be applied bedside. The theoretical base of BIA is that hydrated tissues conduct electricity and different tissues have different electrical conductivity. The impedance characterizes the resistance level of the tissues. BIA provides data about the weighted sum of extra- and intracellular water. Different empirical equations are applied to calculate FFM [15].

Quantitative CT (qCT) and MRI can be also useful methods to measure body composition, precise quantitative and qualitative information can be achieved about body composition, however, due to high-cost, and the need for expert knowledge, its everyday use may be limited. Furthermore, the high dose of radiation is also a disadvantage of CT.

Other methods like total body potassium (using ^{40}K isotope), neutron activation, total body plethysmography, isotope dilution (D_2O dilution or ^{18}O), and MRI are reliable and extremely precise, however, these methods need special equipment with special knowledge and experience, furthermore, are expensive [9].

4. Body composition of patients with IBD

4.1 Crohn's disease compared to healthy population

In a systematic review based on 17 studies, the body composition of 631 CD patients was compared to age-and sex-matched controls [4]. The results were heterogeneous due to variable techniques of body composition measurement, variable study sizes, small control groups, and the lack of standardization of patients according to disease duration, localization, therapy (glucocorticoids), diet, and exercise. BMI was reduced in 37% of patients (n = 233), but it was not statistically different from controls in 63% of patients (n = 398). None of the included studies reported any obese or overweight patients based on BMI. A total of 4% of CD patients were underweight (BMI < 20 kg/m^2).

In addition to BMI, FFM and FM were also compared in patients and healthy controls in the same systematic review [4]. The FM and FFM were not statistically different from controls in 65 and 66% of patients (n = 394, n = 419, respectively). Meanwhile, the FFM was reduced in 28% of CD subjects compared to controls, and 31% of patients with CD (n = 192) had a statistically significant reduction in FM, and 3% were reported to have increased FM relative to controls (n = 20). It is of note, that patients in remission and in relapse were not separated in these comparisons [4].

4.2 Ulcerative colitis

A systematic review of eight studies suggested that the decrease in BMI, FFM, FM are more frequent in patients with CD than in UC patients [4]. The findings of the study including 295 UC patients were heterogenous. BMI was described not statistically different compared to controls in 68% of UC patients (n = 199). Although 20% of UC patients had reduced BMI (n = 60). In contrast to CD, no patients with UC were reported to be underweight.

In this systematic review, FFM was not reported as statistically different compared to controls in 86% of UC patients (n = 256). FFM was reduced compared with healthy controls in 13% of patients studied (n = 39). In 75% of UC patients (n = 220), FM was not found to be statistically different, only 13% of patients experienced reduced FM (n = 39), and 12% of patients had increased FM compared to controls (n = 36) [4].

4.3 Body composition in children with IBD

Lean tissue deficit is also well-documented in children with IBD, especially in the case of CD. Houtto et al. recently published a systematic review of body composition in children with IBD [3]. They included 1461 patients with CD and a total of 264 patients with UC. Growth, FM and FFM were statistically lower in pediatric CD than reference values or healthy cohorts. The results in children with UC were more variable, some studies reported decreased, others found similar body composition parameters as in controls. It is of note, that in a 24-months follow-up study, Thayu et al. reported the body composition of newly diagnosed IBD patients [16]. By the end of the follow-up, patients achieved remission, though LBM was still reduced in girls compared to controls. Dubner et al. also found that the LBM deficit persisted for 12 months [17].

Besides LBM, FM did not differ significantly in pediatric IBD patients when compared with reference or control values, based on the systematic review of Thangarajah et al. [18]. However, patients were receiving concomitant steroid therapy in most of the studies reporting no difference in FM. There is a lack of long-term follow-up studies investigating FM, Boot et al. showed deficits of FM in all the included CD patients with longer disease duration (mean 2.2 years) [19]. Comparing the body composition of children with CD and UC, some studies did not show any difference in deficits in LBM, meanwhile, FM was lower in CD than UC [18].

4.4 Factors influencing body composition

Though it is known that impaired body composition is related to decreased nutrient intake, nutrient loss, and chronic inflammation, there are some factors that influence the body composition in patients with IBD: (1) sex; (2) disease activity; (3) disease duration; (4) disease localization; (5) medication; (6) smoking [4].

Sex: Body composition of healthy women and men are different. In IBD, body composition is associated with sex according to some studies, though the results are heterogenous. According to the systematic review of Bryant et al., two studies reported lower FFM in both males and females compared to controls [4]. Meanwhile, two other studies found deficits in FFM only in males. In addition, Ulivieri et al. reported that females with UC had decreased FFM compared with controls. Regarding FM, the results were heterogenous, and no trends based on sex could be determined [20].

Disease activity: Body composition is associated with disease activity. According to a recent systematic review, BMI of CD patients was lower in the active disease group compared to patients in remission. Moreover, several studies, though with heterogenous methodology, have proved that patients with active disease have lower lean mass and FM than patients in remission [10]. In a systematic review, Thangarajah et al. demonstrated that lean mass deficit is present in children with active CD and half of the children with active UC [18]. Body fat deficits are associated with undernourishment in active CD, however, in remission body fat recovers. It is of note, that lean mass deficit was still reported in at least half of children with IBD in remission [18].

Disease duration: Persisting chronic inflammation has a role in the modulation of body composition due to altered metabolism, however, the results of studies investigating the association between disease duration and body composition, are inconsistent [4, 18]. In case of children, lean mass and FM seem to recover in IBD after diagnosis, however, deficits in lean mass may persist even when the disease is quiescent [18]. Body composition may be not influenced by the disease duration itself, but by the disease course since diagnosis. Initially, most patients with severe disease activity have impaired body composition, later, due to the treatment most patients reach remission, and parallelly body composition is also restored, though partially. Furthermore, patients with refractory disease or recurring disease activity may have persistent changes in their body composition. The studies analyzing this question included heterogenic patients regarding disease course and treatment, so it is not possible to draw any conclusion.

Disease localization: Patients with small intestinal CD experience malabsorption, protein losing enteropathy that has a greater impact on body composition than a short segment inflammation in ulcerative proctitis. Only a few studies analyzed the relationship between disease extension and body composition. Interestingly, FFM did not differ among ileal, ileocolonic, and colonic CD patients in remission [21]. However, FM was significantly lower in CD patients with ileal and ileocolonic disease. Other studies did not report any association between disease localization and body composition [4].

Medication: There are some medications applied in IBD that are related to changes in body composition. One of the most important is glucocorticoids that cause muscle atrophy and lower bone density. Several studies have demonstrated that glucocorticoids decrease bone mineral density in CD patients. Interestingly, in UC patients Ulivieri et al. found a negative correlation between bone density and steroid treatment only in females [22]. Furthermore, patients receiving corticosteroid therapy had lower FFM compared to those without current steroid treatment [23]. The FM was also associated with glucocorticoid treatment, though FM was increased in females, but not in males. In pediatric CD, exclusive enteral nutrition is recommended for induction instead of corticosteroids. During 6-week exclusive enteral nutrition, FFM improved significantly in children with CD, though fat mass did not change [24]. Furthermore, during anti-TNF therapy lean mass increased both in children and in adults, though FM increased only in adults [25, 26].

Smoking: Though smoking is known to be associated with altered body composition and is an important negative prognostic factor in CD, there is only a few data on smoking and body composition in IBD. Most studies record the smoking status of included patients but did not investigate the effect of smoking on body composition. One study found that smoking was a significant predictor of a reduced BMI, FFM, FM in CD [23].

5. Sarcopenia

The term 'sarcopenia' was first applied by Rosenberg to describe the decrease in skeletal muscle mass experienced during aging. According to the recent recommendation of the European Working Group on Sarcopenia in Older People [EWGSOP], sarcopenia can be diagnosed if low lean muscle mass stands together with either low muscle strength or low physical performance [27, 28].

To diagnose sarcopenia according to the current definition, both the mass and the function of the skeletal muscle are to be evaluated. Numerous methods are applied to assess the muscle mass, including BIA, DEXA, CT, and MRI. Functionally, the handgrip strength test with a standard dynamometer or a physical performance test are the gold standard [28].

Recently, the literature demonstrated a correlation between loss of muscle mass in IBD patients with several negative outcomes, such as fatigue, reduced strength, decreased QoL, and increased morbidity [10]. In addition, sarcopenia is considered as a prognostic factor in IBD, like in a variety of other chronic conditions.

The frequency of sarcopenia in IBD varies due to the heterogeneity of the included patient cohorts and the modality used to measure muscle mass. The incidence of sarcopenia was 52% in CD and 37% in UC in a recent systematic review [29]. Notably, in this report, sarcopenia was defined as the reduced muscle mass without functional strength. Data on muscle strength are scarce in IBD patients. Most studies apply hand grip for functional assessments, and they found that IBD patients had lower maximal isometric grip strengths compared to healthy, age,- and sex-matched controls [10]. This was also detected in pediatric CD, but not in UC [30].

Sarcopenia seems to be associated with disease activity via malnutrition and the catabolic effect of inflammation. MRI can be applied to assess sarcopenia. A single cross-sectional MR image at the L3 level for segmentation of skeletal muscle, visceral fat, and subcutaneous adipose tissue areas is used to calculate body composition parameters. The skeletal muscle index [SMI] meaning the ratio of the area of skeletal muscle to the height squared. Labarthe et al. reported that sarcopenia [defined as SMI <38.9 cm^2/m^2 for females and SMI <54.4 cm^2/m^2 in males] was less frequent in patients with inactive CD compared than in patients with active disease [31]. However, 50–60% of patients in remission also suffer from sarcopenia [10].

The distribution of sarcopenia may differ along the body. In a case control study including 23 female UC patients, quadriceps muscle strength was significantly reduced compared with controls and UC patients were significantly slower than controls at the sit-up test. However, the hand grip test did not differ significantly [32]. This finding may indicate assessing muscle functionality with different tests.

To prevent or reduce sarcopenia physical activity with nutritional therapy should be recommended. However, Subramaniam et al. reported an increase in muscle volume and strength at 25 weeks following the commencement of anti-TNF therapy in patients with CD, suggesting that the control of chronic inflammation is also important to overcome sarcopenia [33].

Sarcopenia is certainly an emerging area of interest, given its potential negative effect, and the potential for increased clinical awareness and appropriate management of sarcopenia to improve outcomes and QoL [4].

6. Obesity the impact of obesity in inflammatory bowel disease

Besides the relationship between IBD and undernutrition, there is emerging evidence on the association of obesity with IBD. As obesity rises in the general population, simultaneously the prevalence of obesity is growing in the IBD population. Inflammation is at the core of IBD pathomechanism, and obesity which is a pro-inflammatory status, may also exert an effect on the disease course and severity. It is widely documented that visceral adipose tissue has a role in immunologic dysregulation underlying IBD, known as creeping fat in CD patients. However, data are contradictory regarding the impact of obesity on the frequency of IBD and the disease course [34].

Risk of IBD and obesity First of all, the results of large population-based studies analyzing the association between obesity and IBD are discordant. Based on a recently published pooled analysis of five prospective cohort studies, among 601,009 participants with 10,110,018 person-years of follow-up, 563 incident cases of CD and 1047 incident cases of UC were reported. Obesity was associated with an increased risk of CD compared with normal BMI, meanwhile, no associations were observed between measures of obesity and risk of UC [35].

Frequency of obesity in IBD The rate of obesity in adult CD patients is 8–18% (BMI $\geq$ 30) in Western countries. Studies in pediatric IBD showed that obesity occurred in 23.6% of CD patients and 30.1% of UC patients [36]. In children with newly diagnosed IBD, the frequency of obesity was 2.28% in CD and 5.48% in UC based on BMI [37].

Obesity and disease activity It is also debated whether obesity influences disease activity and disease course. Some studies suggested that obese CD patients have lower disease activity. CD patients with BMI > 30 kg/m^2 were more likely to experience an IBD flare-up than patients with normal BMI. The occurrence of structuring and penetrating complications in obese patients with CD is contradictory. Similarly, overweight (BMI > 25 kg/m^2) UC patients had more frequency of relapse than patients with normal weight. Additionally, obesity was associated with higher rates of colectomy in UC [4, 34].

Response to therapy Obesity is also related to response to therapy. On one hand, through its role in inflammatory processes, obesity manipulates the pharmacodynamics of medical treatments, on the other hand, the accumulated fat mass may also influence the pharmacokinetics of some drugs. Subtherapeutic levels of metabolites of azathioprine were documented approximately two times more in patients with BMI > 25 kg/m^2 or BMI > 30 kg/m^2 than in participants with normal weight [34]. Additionally, a higher BMI has been shown to be associated with the need for dose escalation of adalimumab in CD patients [38]. Furthermore, some studies demonstrated that CD patients on adalimumab or golimumab had higher rates of disease-related hospitalization and operative care compared to infliximab. The explanation for this result is probably the fact that the infliximab dose is adjusted according to weight and intravenously given, whereas adalimumab and golimumab are administered in a fixed dose subcutaneously. Though this was not confirmed in a retrospective study of pediatric IBD patients [34].

Obesity and IBD-related surgeries Higher BMI were also reported to have a negative impact on surgical outcomes in patients with IBD. Intrasurgical complications are mainly related to anatomical difficulties caused by fat tissue [34]. Additionally, obesity may increase the risk of post-surgical morbidity and mortality. According to a recently published meta-analysis, obese patients had longer operative times, higher intra-operative blood loss, longer length of stay, higher wound infection rates, conversion to laparotomy, and higher total postoperative complication rates [39, 40]. Furthermore, post-surgical complications in a nationwide study of hospitalized IBD patients reported that there was no variation in cardiovascular complications, perforations, venous thromboembolism, or death when comparing obese with nonobese patients [34].

Regardless of all controversies, the impact of obesity on the progression of IBDs to further consequences is undeniable [34].

7. Burden of altered body composition

Quality of life: Body composition may affect the quality of life in patients with IBD. As it is known that obese patients have lower QoL compared to healthy populations, and patients with sarcopenia may have lower QoL due to their limited daily activities. Only one study examined this question in adults and did not find any relationship, between altered body composition and QoL, these data are similar to the findings of studies in children [4, 25, 30].

Response to treatment: Body composition can influence treatment response via different mechanisms, such as pharmacokinetics. There are some data on decreased lean mass and response to anti-TNF treatment. Lower skeletal muscle mass was associated with primary non-response to anti-TNF in CD patients [41]. Furthermore, in a retrospective study, CD patients with lower SMM experienced shorter median time to anti-TNF failure defined as treatment escalation, post-induction hospitalization, surgery, and new perianal fistula. In addition, Csontos et al. demonstrated an inverse correlation between FFM index and adalimumab trough levels [42]. Interestingly, not only SMM but also FM is associated with the response to anti-TNF treatment. Lim *et al*. investigated the correlation between body composition measured by CT/MRI scans and trough levels of anti-TNF treatment in a cross-sectional study. They reported higher rate of secondary loss of response to adalimumab in patients with increased total adipose area and an inverse association infliximab trough level and between visceral fat area [43]. Several studies showed that patients on anti-TNF treatment experienced catch-up growth [3]. Data on the impact of body composition on response to new biologicals and small molecules are scarce. However, one study reported that obesity did not influence the efficacy and safety of tofacitinib in UC patients [44].

Prognosis and complications: Changes in body composition has been documented to be associated with complicated CD, increased post-operative complications, and decreased efficacy of medical therapy [10].

8. Recommendation for practice

The association between impaired body composition in IBD such as sarcopenia and increased adiposity and poor clinical outcomes highlights the importance of routine nutritional screening in the care of IBD patients to optimize IBD outcomes. Once realizing impaired body composition, the next challenge is the modulation of body composition through controlling disease activity, nutritional therapy, and physical activity. Excessive FM should also be addressed, and particularly warrants avoidance of steroid therapy.

Since inflammatory cytokines exert a negative effect on appetite and on SMM, one of the first steps to alter lean mass is to control disease activity and achieve remission. It has been demonstrated in a study that during infliximab therapy skeletal muscle mass and muscle strength increased [33].

Nutritional therapy also has a pivotal role in the supportive therapy of IBD patients. In CD patients, concomitant enteral nutrition has been reported to be more effective than infliximab alone. Patients treated with partial enteral nutrition was shown that patients receiving enteral nutrition were less likely to lose response to infliximab compared to controls [45]. Additionally, Gerasimidis et al. found that lean mass improved after the completion of exclusive enteral nutrition [46].

Physical activity with resistance exercise was shown to prevent and even reverse the progression of sarcopenia [47]. Exercise may also contribute to the reduction of the severity of CD and accompanying anorexia while modifying the release of adipokines and ghrelin [12]. Studies on patients with inactive or mildly active CD reported that moderate exercise (walk, yoga) leads to improvement in the quality of life and stress levels [48].

In addition, sarcopenic obesity occurs in some patients, which should be also targeted during the management of IBD patients. Due to the variability of altered body composition experienced in IBD, patients need personalized nutritional intervention.

9. Conclusion

In summary, available data, although heterogeneous, shows that the body composition of patients with IBD may be impaired to a variable extent in comparison with either healthy controls or reference values. However, impaired body composition may not be detected via routine measurement of anthropometrical parameters. The finding of several studies suggests that the prognosis of IBD patients is associated with the alteration of fat and lean mass. The modulation of body composition with nutritional intervention and physical activity can contribute to improve IBD outcomes, including reducing rates of hospitalization, treatment failure, need for surgical intervention and decreasing the incidence of postoperative complications, additionally, it can improve QoL and mental health in IBD patients.

Author details

Katalin E. Müller[1,2]

1 Heim Pal National Pediatric Institute, Budapest, Hungary

2 Faculty of Health Science, Department of Family Care Methodology, Semmelweis University, Budapest, Hungary

*Address all correspondence to: muller.katalin.eszter@gmail.com

References

[1] Cederholm T et al. ESPEN guidelines on definitions and terminology of clinical nutrition. Clinical Nutrition. 2017;**36**(1):49-64

[2] Mehta NM et al. Defining pediatric malnutrition: A paradigm shift toward etiology-related definitions. JPEN Journal of Parenteral and Enteral Nutrition. 2013;**37**(4):460-481

[3] Houttu N et al. Body composition in children with chronic inflammatory diseases: A systematic review. Clinical Nutrition. 2020;**39**(9):2647-2662

[4] Bryant RV et al. Systematic review: Body composition in adults with inflammatory bowel disease. Alimentary Pharmacology & Therapeutics. 2013;**38**(3):213-225

[5] Bilski J et al. The role of physical exercise in inflammatory bowel disease. BioMed Research International. 2014;**2014**:429031

[6] Sylvester FA et al. A two-year longitudinal study of persistent lean tissue deficits in children with Crohn's disease. Clinical Gastroenterology and Hepatology. 2009;**7**(4):452-455

[7] Hill RJ, Davies PS. You look all right to me: Compromised nutritional status in paediatric patients with ulcerative colitis. Journal of Pediatric Gastroenterology and Nutrition. 2013;**56**(4):385-389

[8] Wang ZM, Pierson RN Jr, Heymsfield SB. The five-level model: A new approach to organizing body-composition research. The American Journal of Clinical Nutrition. 1992;**56**(1):19-28

[9] Wells JC, Fewtrell MS. Measuring body composition. Archives of Disease in Childhood. 2006;**91**(7):612-617

[10] Ding NS et al. Systematic review: The impact and importance of body composition in inflammatory bowel disease. Journal of Crohn's & Colitis. 2022;**16**(9):1475-1492

[11] Scaldaferri F et al. Nutrition and IBD: Malnutrition and/or sarcopenia? A practical guide. Gastroenterology Research and Practice. 2017;**2017**:8646495

[12] Bilski J et al. The impact of physical activity and nutrition on inflammatory bowel disease: The potential role of cross talk between adipose tissue and skeletal muscle. Journal of Physiology and Pharmacology. 2013;**64**(2):143-155

[13] Bryant RV et al. Low muscle mass and sarcopenia: Common and predictive of osteopenia in inflammatory bowel disease. Alimentary Pharmacology & Therapeutics. 2015;**41**(9):895-906

[14] Prado CM, Heymsfield SB. Lean tissue imaging: A new era for nutritional assessment and intervention. JPEN Journal of Parenteral and Enteral Nutrition. 2014;**38**(8):940-953

[15] Kyle UG et al. Bioelectrical impedance analysis--part I: Review of principles and methods. Clinical Nutrition. 2004;**23**(5):1226-1243

[16] Thayu M et al. Determinants of changes in linear growth and body composition in incident pediatric Crohn's disease. Gastroenterology. 2010;**139**(2):430-438

[17] Dubner SE et al. Longitudinal assessment of bone density and structure in an incident cohort of children with Crohn's disease. Gastroenterology. 2009;**136**(1):123-130

[18] Thangarajah D et al. Systematic review: Body composition in children with inflammatory bowel disease. Alimentary Pharmacology & Therapeutics. 2015;**42**(2):142-157

[19] Boot AM et al. Bone mineral density and nutritional status in children with chronic inflammatory bowel disease. Gut. 1998;**42**(2):188-194

[20] Ulivieri FM et al. Bone mineral density and body composition in patients with ulcerative colitis. The American Journal of Gastroenterology. 2000;**95**(6):1491-1494

[21] Capristo E et al. Effect of disease localization on the anthropometric and metabolic features of Crohn's disease. The American Journal of Gastroenterology. 1998;**93**(12):2411-2419

[22] Ulivieri FM et al. Bone mineral density and body composition in ulcerative colitis: A six-year follow-up. Osteoporosis International. 2001;**12**(5):343-348

[23] Jahnsen J et al. Body composition in patients with inflammatory bowel disease: A population-based study. The American Journal of Gastroenterology. 2003;**98**(7):1556-1562

[24] Gerasimidis K et al. Impact of exclusive enteral nutrition on body composition and circulating micronutrients in plasma and erythrocytes of children with active Crohn's disease. Inflammatory Bowel Diseases. 2012;**18**(9):1672-1681

[25] Boros KK et al. Body composition, physical activity, and quality of life in pediatric patients with inflammatory bowel disease on anti-TNF therapy-an observational follow-up study. European Journal of Clinical Nutrition. 2023;**77**(3):380-385

[26] Santos J et al. Impact of biological therapy on body composition of patients with Chron's disease. Revista da Associação Médica Brasileira. 2017;**63**:407-413

[27] Rosenberg IH. Sarcopenia: origins and clinical relevance. The Journal of Nutrition. 1997;**127**(5 Suppl):990s-991s

[28] Cruz-Jentoft AJ et al. Sarcopenia: European consensus on definition and diagnosis: Report of the European working group on sarcopenia in older people. Age and Ageing. 2010;**39**(4):412-423

[29] Ryan E et al. Sarcopenia and inflammatory bowel disease: A systematic review. Inflammatory Bowel Diseases. 2019;**25**(1):67-73

[30] Werkstetter KJ et al. Lean body mass, physical activity and quality of life in paediatric patients with inflammatory bowel disease and in healthy controls. Journal of Crohn's & Colitis. 2012;**6**(6):665-673

[31] Labarthe G et al. Magnetic resonance imaging assessment of body composition parameters in Crohn's disease. Digestive and Liver Disease. 2020;**52**(8):878-884

[32] Zaltman C et al. Lower extremity mobility limitation and impaired muscle function in women with ulcerative colitis. Journal of Crohn's & Colitis. 2014;**8**(6):529-535

[33] Subramaniam K et al. Infliximab reverses inflammatory muscle wasting (sarcopenia) in Crohn's disease. Alimentary Pharmacology & Therapeutics. 2015;**41**(5):419-428

[34] Rajabnia M et al. Obesity, a challenge in the management of inflammatory bowel diseases. Immunologic Research. 2022;**70**(6):742-751

[35] Chan SSM et al. Obesity is associated with increased risk of Crohn's disease, but not ulcerative colitis: A pooled analysis of five prospective cohort studies. Clinical Gastroenterology and Hepatology. 2022;**20**(5):1048-1058

[36] Bryant RV et al. Obesity in inflammatory bowel disease: Gains in adiposity despite high prevalence of Myopenia and osteopenia. Nutrients. 1 Sep 2018;**10**(9):1192

[37] Kadenczki O et al. Disease activity is associated with obesity in newly diagnosed Pediatric patients with ulcerative colitis. International Journal of Environmental Research and Public Health. 1 Dec 2022;**19**(23):16091

[38] Bultman E et al. Predictors of dose escalation of adalimumab in a prospective cohort of Crohn's disease patients. Alimentary Pharmacology & Therapeutics. 2012;**35**(3):335-341

[39] Hicks G et al. Outcomes of inflammatory bowel disease surgery in obese versus non-obese patients: A meta-analysis. Techniques in Coloproctology. 2019;**23**(10):947-955

[40] Jiang K et al. Systematic review and meta-analysis: Association between obesity/overweight and surgical complications in IBD. International Journal of Colorectal Disease. 2022;**37**(7):1485-1496

[41] Ding NS et al. The body composition profile is associated with response to anti-TNF therapy in Crohn's disease and may offer an alternative dosing paradigm. Alimentary Pharmacology & Therapeutics. 2017;**46**(9):883-891

[42] Csontos ÁA, Molnár A, Miheller P. Letter: Body surface area and body muscle parameters may influence adalimumab trough levels. Alimentary Pharmacology & Therapeutics. 2015;**41**(7):700

[43] Lim Z et al. The effect of adiposity on anti-tumor necrosis factor-alpha levels and loss of response in Crohn's disease patients. Clinical and Translational Gastroenterology. 2020;**11**(9):e00233

[44] Farraye FA et al. The impact of body mass index on efficacy and safety in the tofacitinib OCTAVE ulcerative colitis clinical programme. Alimentary Pharmacology & Therapeutics. 2021;**54**(4):429-440

[45] Hirai F et al. Effectiveness of concomitant enteral nutrition therapy and infliximab for maintenance treatment of Crohn's disease in adults. Digestive Diseases and Sciences. 2013;**58**(5):1329-1334

[46] Gerasimidis K, McGrogan P, Edwards CA. The aetiology and impact of malnutrition in paediatric inflammatory bowel disease. Journal of Human Nutrition and Dietetics. 2011;**24**(4):313-326

[47] Verdijk LB et al. Skeletal muscle hypertrophy following resistance training is accompanied by a fiber type-specific increase in satellite cell content in elderly men. The Journals of Gerontology. Series A, Biological Sciences and Medical Sciences. 2009;**64**(3):332-339

[48] Loudon CP et al. The effects of physical exercise on patients with Crohn's disease. The American Journal of Gastroenterology. 1999;**94**(3):697-703

Chapter 3

Lactose Intolerance and Small Intestinal Bacterial Overgrowth (SIBO) in Paediatric Patients with Inflammatory Bowel Disease

Sabina Wiecek and Anna Buczynska

Abstract

In recent years, an increase in the incidence of Inflammatory Bowel Disease has been observed, with particular emphasis on Crohn's disease and ulcerative colitis in the paediatric population, also in the youngest age group. Underlying factors are genetic, environmental (including the microbiome) and immunological. Clinical manifestations are very often uncharacteristic, and the clinical picture is dominated by abdominal pain, weight/growth deficiency and/or diarrhoea. Similar symptoms occur in the course of lactose intolerance and small intestinal bacterial overgrowth (SIBO). On the other hand, Inflammatory Bowel Diseases (IBD) seem to favour the onset of SIBO and lactose intolerance. Only the diagnosis of these disease entities ensures appropriate therapeutic management. The manuscript analyses the latest literature on the co-occurrence of these disease entities in patients with IBD—especially Crohn's disease and ulcerative colitis, clinical symptoms, and diagnostic and therapeutic procedures.

Keywords: Crohn's disease, ulcerative colitis, lactose intolerance, small intestinal bacterial overgrowth, children

1. Introduction

In recent years, an increase in the incidence of Inflammatory Bowel Disease has been observed, with particular emphasis on Crohn's disease (CD) and ulcerative colitis (UC) in the paediatric population, also in the youngest age group. Underlying factors are genetic, environmental (including the microbiome) and immunological.

Clinical manifestations are very often uncharacteristic, and the clinical picture is dominated by abdominal pain, weight/growth deficiency and/or diarrhoea. Similar symptoms occur in the course of lactose intolerance and SIBO. On the other hand, Inflammatory Bowel Diseases seem to favour the onset of SIBO and lactose intolerance. Only the diagnosis of these disease entities ensures appropriate therapeutic management [1–6].

2. Lactose intolerance

Lactase is also known as Beta-galactosidase. Its maximum activity can be observed in the descending part of the duodenum and the initial section of the jejunum—on the upper surface of the villi. The activity of lactase can be observed as early as the 12th week of pregnancy, with its peak activity after birth when it is twice as high as in older children. A drop in the lactase activity can be seen from the 2nd-3rd year of life and varies according to ethnicity. Lactase activity is not diet-dependent—the amount of lactose in the diet. It has been stressed that lactose plays an important role in the human body:

- It is a source of energy (human milk contains around 7 g of lactose/100 ml and cow milk around 3.5 g/100 ml);
- It participates in the intestinal regenerative processes;
- It stimulates the growth of acidophiles
- It takes part in calcium metabolism and the absorption of iron
- It impacts the motor activity of the gastrointestinal tract
- It has a low glycaemic index [7–10].

2.1 Epidemiology

The problem of lactose intolerance affects 50% of the adult population of South America and Africa. In the US, it concerns 15% of the white population, 53% of Mexican-Americans and 80% of the black population. In Sicily, lactose intolerance occurs in 70% of adults, in Scandinavia—in 2–5% of the population and in Poland in 20–35% of adults and 20% of school-age children. The meta-analysis on lactose intolerance rates does show a statistically significant increase in prevalence. Adult type-hypolactasia: Among Europeans, two single-nucleotide polymorphisms were described upstream of the LCT–gene: LCT-13910CC and LCT-22018GG. In Europe, the incidence of the LCT 13910CC or 22018GG genotype among healthy adults was 30–40%.

2.2 Clinical manifestations of lactose intolerance

The most common symptoms of lactose intolerance include osmotic diarrhoea, abdominal pain and bloating, rumbling and gurgling. At times, dyspeptic symptoms, nausea and vomiting may occur as well as symptoms of depression caused by the abnormal metabolism of tryptophane. In infants, high levels of acidic metabolites in faeces may irritate the skin of the buttocks [7–10].

Types of lactose intolerance:

1. Congenital alactasia, characterised by a complete lack of lactase activity since birth. The condition is very rare, and only single cases have been reported in the relevant literature. The symptoms are very dramatic and the clinical manifestations are dominated by intense diarrhoea since early infancy—following the introduction of breast-feeding or lactose-containing modified formula—promptly leading to dehydration and a disturbance in the acid–base and electrolyte balance.

Such infants will not tolerate even minute amounts of lactose in their diet. The histopathological examination of the small intestine comes back normal. Only an early diagnosis combined with a lactose-free diet would ensure the survival of such children. A lactose-free diet will have to be adhered to for life.

2. Adult-type hypolactasia—genetically determined—inherited as an autosomal recessive trait. The gene is located on chromosome 2. The activity of lactase is inter-subject variable but never amounts to zero. The activity of the enzyme reduces with age and the time it takes for symptoms to start depends on a number of factors, including the patient's ethnicity. The most common type is a consequence of lactase depletion. The decrease of lactase production starts in the second year of life, although the first symptoms occur in adolescence or adulthood. The structure of the intestinal villi is normal, and organic diseases of the gastrointestinal tract are ruled out.

3. Secondary lactase deficiency. Most commonly observed as a result of damage to/atrophy of the small intestine villi or caused by toxic substances (chemotherapeutics, tetracycline, colchicine), in the course of coeliac disease, food allergy, Crohn's disease, severe giardiasis, radiation-induced intestinal damage and/or post-resection syndromes [7–10].

2.3 Lactose intolerance diagnosis

In most patients, lactose intolerance is diagnosed based on a thorough medical history and the elimination-provocation test using lactose containing products. The following are used additionally in the diagnostics of lactose intolerance:

- The assessment of faecal pH and reducing substances (>0.5%), increase in the amount of lactic acid in stools, increase in osmolity >140mOsmol/l
- Hydrogen breath test after a lactose load—positive test—increased concentration levels of hydrogen >20 ppm during 3-hour examination
- Capillary blood sampling of glucose after an oral lactose load
- The assessment of the activity of lactase in the small bowel mucosa specimen—the procedure is invasive, difficult to perform and not reflecting the full activity of the enzyme in the intestine
- Genetic testing—in the case of adult-type hypolactasia, it does not reflect the actual activity of lactase—it is a gene associated with hypolactasia but the condition may occur at any age. A positive result of the genetic testing does not equal adult-type hypolactasia. However, the test remains valuable in the diagnostics of congenital alactasia.

Some of the factors that affect lactose tolerance include:

a. Increasing tolerance: small amounts, young age, slow emptying of the stomach, high total intestinal lactase and normal intestinal microbiome

b. Reducing tolerance: large amounts, older age, fast emptying of the stomach, low total intestinal activity and abnormal intestinal microbiome [11–17].

<table>
<tr><th>Dairy products rich in lactose (g/100 g)</th><th>Products with average lactose content (g/100 g)</th><th>Dairy products containing a small amount of lactose</th><th>Products with “hidden” lactose</th></tr>
<tr><td rowspan="2">Whole milk (4.9 g)
Fat-free milk (5.3 g)
Buttermilk (4.7 g)
Goat's milk (4.7 g)
Cream flavour, ice cream (4.4 g)
Powdered milk (4.2 g)
Kefir (4.2 g)
Sweet cream (3.9 g)
Ricotta (3.5 g)
Sour cream (ok. 3.5 g)
Cottage cheese (3.2 g)</td><td>Feta cheese (1.4 g)
Butter (0.6–1.1 g)</td><td>Mozzarella (0.7 g)
Cheddar (0.5 g)
Emmentaler and other types of cheese, hard-type cheese, e.g. parmesan, blue cheese, e.g. brie, camembert, gorgonzola: <0.1 g</td><td rowspan="2">Sweets with powdered milk, including chocolate, chocolate bars, confectionary sweets
Ready cake mixes
Bread, rolls, crescent-shaped rolls (a full-butter croissant contains on average 48 g of butter so approx. 3 g of lactose)
Sauces, including ready ones, soups, puree and margarine</td></tr>
<tr><td colspan="2">Yoghurts: similar to kefirs and depending on the production process (the fermentation, the addition of milk powder) may contain from 0.5 (very rarely) to 4.5 of lactose. The most common products available on the market on average contain 3.3 g/100 g</td></tr>
</table>

Table 1.
The content of lactose in differed foodstuffs.

2.4 Treatment of lactose intolerance

The primary treatment of lactose intolerance is a diet aimed at reducing the intake of this disaccharide. Some of the products rich in lactose include sweet milk, cream and ice-cream. Fermented products like kefir, yoghurt and probiotic-enriched foods are recommended in patients with diagnosed lactose intolerance. In the cases when it is impossible to exclude lactose-containing products, pharmacological supplementation with lactase is recommended. It is important to take into account that lactose is a component of certain medication and foodstuffs.

The amount of lactose varies in the different types of dairy products and there is a large content of “hidden” lactose in many products not derived from dairy. **Table 1** presents the summary of safe and not-recommended foodstuffs in lactose intolerance [8–10, 18, 19].

Ultimately, whether the clinical symptoms occur or not after a lactose-containing meal depends not only on the amount of lactose but also on the content of the whole meal, so the amount of protein and fat.

3. Small intestinal bacterial overgrowth

This is an abnormal, excessive growth of commensal bacterial in the small intestine, leading to abnormalities in the digestion and absorption of mainly fats and vit. B12. The excessive growth mainly involves the following bacteria: *Escherichia coli, Enterococcus spp., Klebsiella pneumoniae.* Dysbiosis is an imbalance in the intestinal microbial community leading to the loss of probiotics and the appearance of pathogenic strains. The type and proportions of the bacteria (enterotypes) take shape with age and the lifestyle and ensure the homeostasis of the gastrointestinal tract. Bacteriocins produced by probiotic bacteria with their bacteriostatic or bactericidal properties against sensitive pathogens modify the composition of the intestinal microbiota. The growth of the pathogenic bacteria is linked to the increase in the concentration levels of toxic and genotoxic bacterial metabolites not only in the intestine but also in the general circulation. Toxins induce mutations and by doing so they impact the transduction of the intracellular signals. The deconjugation of bile acids contributes to the maldigestion of fats and the production of the lithocholic acid, which may be toxic for enterocytes. The damage to the intestinal barrier leads to the translocation of the bacteria from the intestinal lumen to the surrounding tissues, lymph glands and the circulatory system. The enterotoxins reaching the liver are strong activators of the T CD8 cytotoxic lymphocytes, which play a role in the fibrogenesis.

The first study by Faber describing the link between pernicious anaemia and intestinal narrowing was published in 1897. In 1939, Barker and Hummel put forward a hypothesis that there was a link between pernicious anaemia and small intestinal bacterial overgrowth. The microbiome plays a role not only in the pathogenesis of the disorders of the gastrointestinal tract but also of the respiratory tract, the circulatory system, the endocrine system, the urinary system and/or the osteoarticular system. It affects the functioning of the central nervous system; it impacts the mood and the processes of perception [17, 20–23].

Non-pathogenic intestinal bacteria impact the development of the immune system, the morphology of the intestinal villi and the intestinal crypts and the motor activity.

In the clinical studies of healthy persons, SIBO is present in 0–20%.

Some of the mechanisms that protect from the development of small intestinal bacterial overgrowth include the following:

- Low-pH gastric juice
- The presence of pancreatic juice, which contains bactericidal enzymes (proteolytic and lipolytic)
- The normal motor activity of the small intestine
- The presence of mucosa lining the intestinal epithelium
- The gut mucosal immune system—secretory IgA, the Paneth cells
- Antibacterial property of bile
- Anatomical barrier between the colon and the small intestine—the ileocecal valve [17, 20–23].

Factors contributing to the occurrence of small intestinal bacterial overgrowth are presented below (**Table 2**) [17, 20–26].

It has to be remembered that the chronic use of proton pump inhibitors is an independent factor in the development of SIBO (decrease in the population of Bacteroides and increase in Firmicutes), which may lead to an increase in Clostridioides difficile.

Factors influencing the risk of developing SIBO	
Anatomical anomalies	**The presence of intestinal diverticula, intestinal fistula, intestinal strictures**
Post-surgical lesions	lleocecal valve resection, gastroenterostomy bypass, Roux-en-Y-type surgeries, post-operative adhesions
Medication affecting the motor activity of the gastrointestinal tract	opiodis, anticholinergics medication used in the treatment of diarrhoea/constipation
Reduced secretion of gastric juice	Conducted gastrectomy, autoimmune gastritis, chronic use of proton pump inhibitors
Insufficient digestive enzymes/bile acids	Cystic fibrosis, chronic pancreatitis, cirrhosis (PPC, PBC)
Disorders of the motor activity of the small intestine	Bowel inflammatory diseases, coeliac disease, radiation enteritis, diabetes, amyloidosis, scleroderma, intestinal pseudo-obstruction, gastroparesis drug-induced (opioids, anticholinergics)
Immunodeficiencies	HIV, congenital immunodeficiency (primary hypogammaglobulinaemia, immunosuppressive therapy)
Inflammatory	Non-specific inflammatory bowel diseases
Infections	Infections of the gastrointestinal tract
Metabolic	Diabetes
Dietary	High-fat, high-carbohydrate and low-fibre diet
Others	Irritable bowel syndrome

Table 2.
Factors contributing to the occurrence of small intestinal bacterial overgrowth.

Small intestinal bacterial overgrowth leads to many serious complications, some of which include the following:

1. Abnormalities in the metabolism of fatty acids—fat digestion disorders - > steatorrhea, and malabsorption of fat-soluble vitamins

2. B12-deficiency anaemia

3. Secondary malabsorption syndromes

4. Disaccharidase deficiency and as a result of the abnormalities in their digestion and absorption

5. Increased absorption of antigens through damaged mucosa (immune complexes).

3.1 Microbiome and other diseases

There are studies dedicated to the impact of the changes to the microbiome on the following comorbidities:

DOI: http://dx.doi.org/10.5772/intechopen.1003061

- obesity and metabolic syndrome
- diabetes mellitus
- dyslipidaemia
- food allergies
- autoimmune diseases
- coeliac disease
- inflammatory bowel diseases
- irritable bowel syndrome

3.1.1 Epidemiology of small intestinal bacterial overgrowth

Accurate data concerning the occurrence of SIBO in the European and global population is unknown. SIBO affects around 50% of the patients who underwent gastrojejunostomy and vagotomy, 5% of the patients after vagotomy and pyloroplasty and 2–10% of those with autonomic diabetic neuropathy. There is no data concerning the paediatric population.

3.1.2 Clinical manifestations of small intestinal bacterial overgrowth

Very often the clinical manifestations of SIBO are highly non-specific and of little use in the diagnostic process. The more proximal section of the small intestine is affected by SIBO, the more severe the course of the disease is.

The clinical picture is dominated by the following:

- abdominal bloating/feeling full/excessive flatulence
- abdominal pain
- diarrhoea/constipation
- nausea/vomiting
- dyspeptic symptoms
- heartburn, regurgitation
- tiredness
- insufficient body weight
- oedema (intestinal loss of protein)
- ataxia, peripheral neuropathy

There is a link between the occurrence of irritable bowel syndrome (IBS) and of small intestinal bacterial overgrowth. Undoubtedly, the population of the bacteria present in the intestinal lumen plays a role—through the metabolic processes; the population of the bacteria in the intestinal mucosa—through the activation of immunological interactions with the host and the induction of persistent moderate inflammation. A decrease in the number of Lactobacillus and Bifidobacterium and an increase in the numbers of Clostridium and Enterobacteriaceae are observed. The bacteria forming the intestinal ecosystem of patients with IBS show little stability and are susceptible to significant malfunctions in the case of even mildly intensive factors such as stress, a diet high in animal-based saturated fats and synthetic carbohydrates, surgical procedures, non-steroidal anti-inflammatory drugs, proton pump inhibitors, H2 blockers, prokinetics and antibiotics.

3.1.3 Diagnostics of small intestinal bacterial overgrowth

A hydrogen and methane breath test is commonly used in the diagnostics of the condition. The cells of the human body do not produce methane or hydrogen in their gas forms. Their presence in the exhaled air indicates an increased metabolism of carbohydrates in the intestinal lumen. The production of gas in the intestinal lumen in the course of SIBO varies and depends on the volume and the types of the bacterial colonising the small intestine as well as the amount of carbohydrates in the lumen of the intestine and the intestinal capability of their absorption. According to NASPGHAN, a heathy body contains between 30 and 100 ml of gas in the lumen of the intestine and it is mainly hydrogen, carbon dioxide, methane as well as smaller amounts of oxygen, nitrogen, hydrogen sulphide and ammonia. Enterobacteriaceae may also produce trace amounts of indole and its derivative—skatole, the so-called odorous gases. There are four main sources of intestinal gases. These are as follows: those swallowed with food, chemical reactions forming in the lumen of the intestine, blood diffusion and the metabolism of the intestinal bacteria. The last mechanism in the sole source of the origin of hydrogen and methane is used in the breath tests techniques. Anaerobic bacteria, which inhabit the large intestine in physiological conditions and the small intestine also in non-physiological conditions, cause the fermentation of undigested carbohydrates, and following the diffusion of thus resulting gases into the blood and their transport to the lungs—an increase in their concentration levels in the alveolar air [12–14, 16, 17, 26–28].

There is no single diagnostic test that would allow for the conclusive diagnosis of SIBO. Very often it is a good response to an empirical antibacterial treatment that acts as a confirmation.

1. Lactulose hydrogen breath test

    - 10 g of lactulose-disaccharide non-absorbable in the small intestine, water-soluble and subject to fermentation
    - Metabolised by gut microbiota ->hydrogen produced in the reaction
    - (+) test—increased concentration levels of hydrogen >20 ppm in the 90th minute after the oral administration of lactulose

2. Glucose hydrogen breath test—recommended. Following the oral administration of glucose and as a result of the fermentation processes, hydrogen is produced. An increase in the concentration levels of hydrogen >20 ppm after glucose load is considered a positive result.

3. Quantitative and qualitative culture of jejunal aspirates—the gold standard (important: technical challenges of sample collection, the risk of sample contamination, possibility of false-negative results). Quantitative and qualitative microbial investigation of duodenal or jejunal aspirates are considered the gold standard in the diagnostics of SIBO but techniques of aseptic sample collection are not standardised; during the endoscopy of the upper section of the gastrointestinal tract 3–5 ml of the content is aspirated and placed in aerobic and anaerobic conditions in a growth medium—SIBO is confirmed at the value of $\geq 10^3$ CFU/ml of the aspirate; the most common strains include *Escherichia*, *Shigella*, *Aeromonas*, *Pseudomonas*.

4. The PCR analysis of the contents of the jejunum.

Table 3 shows the doses of the substrates used in hydrogen breath tests.

There is a consensus in the diagnostics of SIBO that glucose seems to be more reliable than lactulose, which results from a greater probability of obtaining a false-positive result with lactulose because it accelerates the peristalsis.

As regards the assessment of the concentration of methane in the exhaled air this is recommended because around 1/3 of the European population is colonised with methane-producing microbiota such as *Methanobrevibacter smithii*. Its presence lowers the result of the hydrogen test because of the use of hydrogen as a substrate in the production of methane. Therefore, it is considered one of the reasons for a false-negative result. The colonisation of children with methanogenic bacteria is smaller; however, the incidence may be comparable to the adult population.

An increase of over 20 ppm in the concentration levels of hydrogen and of over 10 ppm of that of methane is considered a positive result. The starting—so before the load—concentration level of hydrogen in the exhaled air should be less than 10 ppm (according to ESPGHAN it is 7+/−5 ppm). If the obtained values are >10 ppm, the test should be stopped so the patient should not be given the tested disaccharide.

Substrate	Aim of the diagnostics	ESNM—adults	ESNM—children	EPGHAN/ NASPGHAN
		2021		2022
Glucose	SIBO	50 g in 250 ml of water	2 g/kg max. 50 g in 200–250 ml of water	50 g or 1 g/kg
Lactulose		10–20 g in 250 ml of water	10–20 g in 100–200 ml of water	10 g
Lactose	Lactose intolerance	25-50 g in the diagnostics of lactose malabsorption, 25 g in the diagnostics of lactose intolerance	0.5-2 mg/kg (max.25-50 g) in the volume corresponding to the 10–20% solution	50 g or 1 g/kg

Table 3.
Doses of the substrates used in breath tests.

Causes of questionable results of breath tests		
Invalid collection on an empty stomach	**False-positive results in intolerance testing**	**False-negative tests in intolerance testing**
Diet rich in non-absorbable carbohydrates the day before the test	SIBO	Lack of hydrogen-generating microbiota (10% of the population)—may be determined with a lactulose test because lactulose is not absorbed in healthy people. Medication—antibiotics and/or macrogol. Lack of cooperation with the patient (if the test is performed in a standard way so without a valved mask)
Insufficient oral hygiene	Significantly accelerated OCTT	Significantly prolonged OCTT (if fermentation occurs once the measurements have been taken)

Table 4.
Causes of questionable results of breath tests.

ESNM recommends that if the result is ≥15 ppm on an empty stomach, the patient should be asked to rinse their mouth with water and the test can then be re-taken [12–14, 16, 17, 26–28]. **Table 4** presents the causes of questionable results of breath tests.

The treatment of SIBO involves three stages:

1. Remission induction therapy—lasts between 5 days and 1 month—repetitive cycles (optimum 14 days)

2. Sustaining of remission

3. The treatment of/the modification of the factors underlying the bacterial growth

Rifaximin forms the basis of the treatment. It is an antibiotic and a eubiotic—it acts as a modulator of the intestinal microenvironment. Rifaximin has antibacterial, anti-inflammatory properties—it modulates the immune response of the host, lowers the IL-6 and alpha TNF and binds the pregnane X receptor—PXR. It also modulates the activity of the intestinal microbiome (the metabolism, the binding and the virulence). Additionally, it hinders the bacterial interaction with the body and the activation of its immune response. Rifaximin is used in the dose of 800–1650 mg/day for 10–14 days. The TARGET 1, TARGET 2 and TARGET 3 studies of patients with IBS have shown the disappearance of symptoms in 40.7% and a reduction in bloating in 40.2% (NNT-10.1). About 83–86% of patients had a negative result of the control hydrogen breath test. The eradication of the bacteria and the disappearance of symptoms were observed in 70% of patients. Rifaximin showed its antibacterial effects against *E.coli, Klebsiella spp., Enterobacter spp. and Enterococcus faecalis* [17, 20–23].

The meta-analysis of 32 clinical studies involving a total of 1331 patients showed that the proportion of the eradication of SIBO following the administration of rifaximin and confirmed with breath test was 72.9%, and the withdrawal of symptoms was confirmed in 67.7% of patients with SIBO. The daily recommended dose of rifaximin for adults is 1600 mg/day for 14 days. In the case of the recurrence of SIBO, the treatment with rifaximin may be cyclical with 30-day intervals between the cycles [17, 20–23].

SIBO is characterised as relapsing because after receiving the first successful dose of antibiotics, approximately 44% of patients suffer from the same symptoms again after 9 months. Based on the severity of the symptoms and their rapidity of return, patients usually need to follow a regimen of rotating different antibiotics [17, 20–23].

OTHER ANTIBIOTICS used in the treatment of SIBO

- Ciprofloxacin
- Metronidazole
- Doxycycline
- Amoxicillin
- Neomycin

PROBIOTICS- even though the use of antibiotics in the treatment of SIBO may seem illogical, experiments conducted on rats indicate that probiotics may act as prokinetic agents. The meta-analysis investigating the use of probiotics in SIBO showed a decrease in the production of hydrogen (OR 1.61; 95% CI: 1.19–2.17). However, the studies included in the meta-analysis involved small groups of patients, different preparations of probiotics were used, and different final outcomes were assessed. In a recent randomised study, it has been shown that probiotics may cause SIBO and lactic acidosis, and may trigger excessive flatulence and bloating. These symptoms disappeared once the probiotic was stopped and an antibiotic was introduced.

Undoubtedly, probiotics have a beneficial effect on the intestinal microbiome, they modulate the balance between saprophytes and pathogenic bacteria, and they restore the microbiological homeostasis of the intestines. Some probiotics have the ability to stimulate the production of mucin by increasing the expression of the MUC2 genes. Probiotics may be identified based on their ability to colonise the intestinal mucosa, which, in the future, may facilitate targeted therapies, according to the clinical needs. Probiotics may increase the effectiveness of the antibiotic therapy, for example, *Lactobacillus casei*. There is some evidence suggesting that during a prolonged therapy with proton pump inhibitors the probiotic bacteria *Bacillus subtilis* and *Enterococcus faecium* may be effective in the therapy of SIBO. However, controlled, double-blind clinical studies are needed to confirm which probiotic strains are effective, their doses and the duration of therapy. Therefore, the ACG experts concluded that there is no data justifying the use of probiotics in the treatment of SIBO [17, 20–23].

FAECAL TRANSPLANT The data concerning the effectiveness of faecal microbiota transplantation in patients with SIBO is scant and casuistical. Currently, it is not recommended in the treatment of SIBO. Additionally, recently there have been warnings about the risk of transferring multidrug-resistant bacteria during the procedure. There are no grounds for routine faecal microbiota transplantation when treating SIBO.

3.1.4 Diet and SIBO

The main dietary modification in SIBO is the reduction in the intake of fermentable foods and those low in fibre, polyols, and fermenting sweeteners such as sucralose. Also, prebiotics, for example inulin, should be avoided. The introduction of the

FODMAP diet, so one with small amounts of fermentable oligo-, di- and monosaccharides, and polyols. However, this diet should only be used for a limited time—from 4 to 6 weeks.

Elemental diets may be a safe and effective alternative for antibiotics—for those patients not tolerating antibiotics or not responding to them. The nutrients are absorbed in the initial sections of the small intestine and do not reach the bacteria in the further sections of the intestine. Such therapy should last at least 2 weeks.

Undoubtedly, the following support the treatment:

- Regular meals
- Avoiding large volumes of meals
- Reducing the fat content in the diet
- Reducing the content of foods which cause bloating

The treatment of the primary disease is of paramount importance in the following:

- Inflammatory bowel Diseases
- Coeliac disease
- Diverticulosis
- Connective-tissue diseases—autoimmune disease (lupus, scleroderma)
- Diabetes mellitus
- Adhesive disease

SIBO complications—deconjugation of bile acids leading to impaired digestion of fats → steatorrhea and abnormal absorption of fat-soluble vitamins; intra-intestinal decomposition of proteins by the bacteria → abnormal absorption of amino acids; vitamin B_{12} deficiency → megaloblastic anaemia; damage to the intestinal villi and defective digestion of disaccharides → the lowering of the pH of the intestinal contents, excessive concentration of gases and bloating; excessive breaking down of proteins and urea with the production of ammonia → conducive for the development of encephalopathy in patients with liver failure; increased absorption of bacterial antigens into the bloodstream.

SIBO prevention:

- avoiding prolonged therapy with proton pomp inhibitors
- concurrent administration of IPP and probiotics, e.g. Bacillus subtilis, Enterococcus faecium
- avoiding unnecessary antibiotic therapy
- the treatment of the primary disease [17, 18, 20–23].

4. Small intestinal bacterial overgrowth and inflammatory bowel disease

The composition of the gastrointestinal microbiota has a strong impact on the homeostasis of the entire organism. Imbalances of this part of the body can lead to the occurrence of many conditions and diseases. The intestinal microbiota is an essential element with regard to IBD. The gut microbiota is different in patients with Crohn's disease where the disease is manifested in the colon and ileum. Lactose consumption helps maintain the balance of gut microbiota composition. Moreover, lactose contributes to the development of Bifidobacterium and other lactic acid bacteria. The change in the microbial population of the gastrointestinal tract can lead to inflammation. SIBO in patients with IBD may have clinical significance as it may contribute to the pathogenesis, symptom development, malabsorption with consequent malnutrition, altered drug metabolism and poor response to therapy [4, 17, 29–32].

According to various reports, the frequency of SIBO occurrence is between 18 and 30% for Crohn's disease and 14 and 17.8% for ulcerative colitis when the hydrogen breath test is used as a diagnostic method. Andrei et al. showed the prevalence of SIBO in patients with Crohn's disease—overall, of the entire group of patients screened, SIBO was present in 30.77% of patients with CD—in particular in the patients with strictures, extensive lesions and advanced perianal lesions. Prevalence of SIBO in patients with ulcerative colitis was 19.4%. Distribution according to the Montreal classification: 28.5% with extended colitis, 25% with left-sided colitis and no patient with ulcerative proctitis [24]. Ghoshal in his study showed that patients with IBD had a higher risk of SIBO than healthy controls. SIBO was commoner among Crohn's disease than ulcerative colitis. The factors associated with the presence of SIBO among patients with IBD included female gender, low serum total protein, albumin and prior surgical treatment for IBD [4]. This data was confirmed by Ricci et al. who proved that SIBO is a highly prevalent condition in patients with Crohn's disease [33]. Wanzl has shown that an increased amount of SIBO was found in IBD patients and was especially more frequent in patients with Crohn's disease than in those with ulcerative colitis. In patients with ulcerative colitis, SIBO rates were not different to patients with other gastrointestinal diseases investigated. In active IBD positive SIBO was detected more often [31]. Shah has conducted a systematic review with meta-analysis—the dataset included 11 studies (1175 adult patients with IBD and 407 controls)—all using the breath test for the diagnosis of SIBO. The proportion of SIBO in IBD patients was 22.3% [32]. However, Wei believes that patients with SIBO had a 2.27-fold elevated risk of clinical relapse compared to those without SIBO [34].

The risk factors that were identified as associated with the presence of SIBO in IBD patients are as follows:

- extended ulcerative colitis
- perianal and ileocolonic involvement in Crohn's disease
- fibrostenosing forms of Crohn's disease
- post-operative condition—postoperative absence of the ileocecal valve
- dysfunctions of the motor activity of the gastrointestinal tract
- abdominal fistulas
- drugs used in treatment—immunosuppressants [34, 35].

However, Sanchez-Montes believes that immunosuppressants and/or biological drugs do not induce SIBO in inactive CD. Fistulising disease pattern and meteorism are associated with SIBO [36].

5. Lactose intolerance and inflammatory bowel disease

The clinical symptoms of non-specific inflammatory bowel diseases and lactose intolerance may very often be similar and manifest themselves as abdominal pain, stomach gurgling, bloating and increased flatulence and/or belching. Sometimes, the distinction between the two conditions may be very difficult if it is only based on the clinical manifestations. On the other hand, differentiating the symptoms of the inflammatory bowel disease from symptoms of food intolerance is important to avoid the overtreatment of IBD-related intestinal inflammation, given its associated adverse effects. It is a condition with an inability to digest and absorb lactose and may occur in IBD patients because of the resulting changes in the structure and function of the GI tract related to the chronic inflammatory state of IBD [1–3, 37–41].

The largest meta-analysis by Szilagyi et al. included 17 studies and 1935 IBD patients. The risk of lactose maldigestion was reported to be higher among IBD patients than the controls. In subgroup analysis, the risk of lactose maldigestion was only significant for Crohn disease but not ulcerative colitis patients compared another study [42]. Mishkin reported that lactose intolerance prevalence in ulcerative colitis patients was more likely to follow the normal population, whereas Crohn's disease patients had prevalence beyond the ethnic risk [43]. The additional risk in Crohn's disease and intolerance lactose:

- Ethnic risk
- Location of the disease—the small bowel having the highest risk
- Coexistence small intestinal bacterial overgrowth
- Surgical treatment
- Exacerbation/acute phase disease
- Increased small bowel transit time
- Immunosuppressive therapy

The significance of decreased duodenal lactase levels in some patients with inflammatory bowel disease remains controversial.

Eadala et al., in their examination of 165 IBD patients with CC13910 genotype, reported that sensitivity to lactose occurs in a high percentage of patients in remission. They highlighted the importance of a thorough consideration of lactose malabsorption in IBD patients because of their similar symptomatology [3].

Research by Jasielska et al. indicated that lactose intolerance occurred in 23.2% of children with ulcerative colitis and 22.6% of those with CD. Secondary lactose intolerance in IBD was diagnosed in 6.7% of patients and its occurrence was not dependent on such factors as location, activity and duration of the disease or the number of relapses in the past [5]. On the other hand, Pawłowska et al. reported that lactose intolerance affected about 30% of children with IBD. In terms of IBD about 40% of patients with active IBD and about 33% of those in remission avoided products with lactose [10]. In his study, Tirpitz reported lactose intolerance in 46.9% of the patients with Crohn's disease compared to 16.6% of those from the control group. A very high incidence rate of lactose intolerance was observed in the patients with the active form of the disease (CDAI>150)—83.3% and a long duration of the disease. Unlike other scientists, he did not show a correlation with the scope of the lesions and the condition after bowel resection [44]. Kirschner et al. were not able to show any statistically significant difference in the prevalence of lactose intolerance in children and adolescents with ulcerative colitis and Crohn's disease. Involvement of the terminal ileum, disease activity and previous surgery have been discussed as determinants of intolerance lactose. He believed that the pathomechanism of lactose intolerance in patients with Crohn's disease is not fully understood. Lactose maldigestion may be influenced by bacterial overgrowth and increased small bowel transit time [38]. Park et al. performed enzyme assays on jejunal biopsies. He did not find any increased prevalence of lactose intolerance in patients with inflammatory bowel disease [39]. In contrast, Dunnee et al. observed a significant reduction of lactase and other disaccharidases in mucosal biopsies from the proximal jejunum in Crohn's disease patients. In patients with ulcerative colitis patients did not differ from the healthy control group [12]. In our studies (Wiecek and al.) assessing the activity of disaccharidases in the small intestine biopsy in children with IBD, a decreased activity of lactase was found in 33% of patients with Crohn's disease and in 20% children with ulcerative colitis [45]. On the other hand, Pfefferkorn et al. did not show an increased incidence of decreased lactase activity in the intestine biopsies of patients with IBD in relation to healthy control [40]. Also, Nardone concluded the prevalence of lactose intolerance in IBD patients did not differ from that of control. Despite presenting suggestive symptoms, about 1/3 of IBD patients are not lactose intolerant, thus not needing "*a priori*" elimination diet [37].

The role of dairy foods in inflammatory bowel disease has been controversial and confounded by the phenotypic divide of lactase status in the adult population. In several polish studies, the incidence of the LCT-13910CC genotype associated with ATH in healthy people was estimated at 30–31.5%. It is suggested that lactose intolerance in inflammatory bowel disease is determined by ethnicity in most cases of ulcerative colitis and Crohn's disease. Buning et al. in Germany did not find differences in the incidence of LCT-22018GG and LCT-13910CC genotypes between patients with IBD, their first-degree relatives and healthy volunteers [2]. Nolan et al. demonstrated with a large group of patients that T-allele in locus LCT-13910, responsible for lactase persistence, occurs more often in patients with Crohn's disease [29]. On the other hand, Elguezabal also did not prove any connection between the genotype LCT-13910CC and inflammatory bowel diseases [35].

It has to be remembered that unnecessary elimination of dairy products from the diet may aggravate these deficiencies. Many IBD patients are already undernourished, especially those with uncontrolled disease or in acute flares; restrictive diets can further worsen their malnutrition. Avoiding dairy products and its associated long-term effects on bone density contributes to the increasing rates of osteoporosis among IBD patients, who are already at an increased risk, particularly those on chronic steroid or immunosuppressants. It is important to evaluate IBD patients to lactose intolerance before subjecting them to a lactose-restricted diet, given its potential adverse effects.

6. Summary

When objective evidence of active inflammation does not correlate with the persistent symptoms in IBD patients, clinicians should consider other disease with alternative pathophysiological mechanisms presenting with functional gastrointestinal symptoms, small intestine bacterial overgrowth and/or food intolerance (e.g. lactose intolerance). Differentiating the symptoms of IBD-related inflammatory changes from symptoms of non-IBD diseases is important to avoid the overtreatment of IBD-related intestinal inflammation, given their associated adverse effects.

The comparison between the clinical picture of lactose intolerance, small intestinal bacterial overgrowth and inflammatory bowel disease is shown in **Table 5**.

Parameter	Lactose intolerance	Small intestinal bacterial overgrowth	Inflammatory bowel disease
Pathogenesis	Genetic background Lactase deficiency Lactose maldigestion	Dysfunction of the intestinal microbiome Dysfunction of the motor activity of the gastrointestinal tract	Genetic factors Immunological factors Environmental factors
Clinical symptoms	Diarrhoea/constipation Bloating Abdominal pain Nausea	Diarrhoea/constipation Bloating Abdominal pain Nausea Loss of body weight/difficulty getting weight Loss of appetite Anaemia	Diarrhoea/constipation Bloating Abdominal pain Nausea Loss of body weight/difficulty getting weight Loss of appetite Gastrointestinal bleeding Fever Anaemia
Abnormalities in the laboratory tests	No	Anaemia Hypoproteinaemia B12 deficiency	Anaemia Elevated parameters of inflammation High concentration of calprotectin in stools
Diagnostics	Elimination and challenge lactose Hydrogen breath test Lactose/methane breath test The presence of faecal reducing substances Genetic tests The assessment of lactase activity in mucosal biopsies	Lactulose/glucose hydrogen/methane breath test Quantitative/qualitative assessment of the intestinal flora	Colonoscopy/gastroscopy with the histopathological assessment of the samples MRI enterography
Treatment	Elimination diet Supplementation with lactase	Antibiotics-Rifaximin Diet therapy-reduction of FOODMAP Faecal transplantation	Diet therapy-Modulife IBD Immunosuppressing treatment • mesalazine • glucocorticoids • biological treatment • methotrexate • azathioprine Surgical treatment

Parameter	Lactose intolerance	Small intestinal bacterial overgrowth	Inflammatory bowel disease
Complications	Worsening of the quality of life	Anaemia Malnutrition	Anaemia Malnutrition Strictures, Abdominal fistulas, enterocutaneous fistulas, perianal lesions
Prognosis	Life-long condition from the onset of symptoms	Very high risk of recurrence	Chronic, progressive disease with periods of remissions and relapses

Table 5.
The comparison between the clinical picture of lactose intolerance, small intestinal bacterial overgrowth and inflammatory bowel disease.

Author details

Sabina Wiecek* and Anna Buczynska
Department of Paediatrics, Medical University of Silesia, Katowice, Poland

*Address all correspondence to: sabinawk@wp.pl

References

[1] Asfari M, Sarmini M, Kendrick K, et al. Association between inflammatory bowel disease and lactose intolerance: Fact or fiction. The Korean Journal of Gastroenterology. 2020;**76**(4):185-190. DOI: 10.4166/kjg.2020.76.4.185

[2] Buning C, Ockenga J, Kruger S, et al. The C/C-13910 and G/G 22018 genotypes for adult -type hypolactasia are not associated with inflammatory bowel disease. Scandinavian Journal of Gastroenterology. 2003;**38**(5):538-542

[3] Eadala P, Matthews S, Waud J, et al. Association of lactose sensitivity with inflammatory bowel disease-demonstrated by analysis of genetic polymorphism, breath gases and symptoms. Alimentary Pharmacology & Therapeutics. 2011;**34**:735-746

[4] Ghoshal U, Yadav A, Fatima B, et al. Small intestinal bacterial overgrowth in patients with inflammatory bowel disease: A case- control study. Indian Journal of Gastroenterology. 2022;**41**(1):96-103

[5] Jasielska M, Grzybowska-Chlebowczyk U. Lactose malabsorption and lactose intolerance in children with inflammatory bowel diseases. Gastroenterology Research and Practice. 2019;**2019**:2507242. DOI: Doi.org/10.1155/2019/2507242

[6] Klaus J, Spaniol U, Adler G, et al. Small intestinal bacterial overgrowth mimicking acute flare as a pitfall in patients with Crohn's disease. BMC Gastroenterology. 2009;**9**:61. DOI: 10.1186/1471-230X-9-61

[7] Pironi L, Callegari C, Cornia G, et al. Lactose malabsorption in adult patients with Crohn's disease. The American Journal of Gastroenterology. 1988;**83**:1267-1271

[8] Kluch M, Socha-Banasiak A, Paczes K, et al. The role of disaccharidases in the digestion- diagnosis and significance of their deficiency in children and adults. Polski Merkuriusz Lekarski. 2020;**49**(286):275-278

[9] Harvey L, Ludwig T, Qian HA, Hock Q, et al. Prevalence, cause and diagnosis of lactose intolerance in children aged 1-5 years: A systematic review of 1995-2015 literature. Asia Pacific Journal of Clinical Nutrition. 2018;**27**(1):29-46. DOI: 10.6133/apjcn.022017.05

[10] Pawłowska K, Umławska W, Iwańczak B. Prevalence of lactose malabsorption and lactose intolerance in pediatric patients with selected gastrointestinal diseases. Advances in Clinical and Experimental Medicine. 2015;**24**(5):863-871

[11] Lember M. Hypolactasia: A common enzyme deficiency leading to lactose malabsorption and intolerance. Polish Archives of Internal Medicine. 2012;**122**:160-164

[12] Dunne W, Cooke W, Alen R. Enzymatic and morphometric evidence for Crohn's disease as a diffuse lesion of the gastrointestinal test. Gut. 1977;**18**:290-294

[13] Eisenmann A, Amann A, Said M, Datta B, et al. Implementation and interpretation of hydrogen breath tests. Journal of Breath Research. 2008;**2**(4):046002. DOI: 10.1088/1752-7155/2/4/046002

[14] Gasbarrini A, Corazza GR, Gasbarrini G, 1st Rome H2-Breath

Testing Consensus Conference Working Group. Methodology and indications of H_2-breath testing in gastrointestinal diseases: The Rome consensus conference. Alimentary Pharmacology & Therapeutics. 2009;**30**(29 Suppl 1):1-49. DOI: 10.1111/j.1365-2036.2009.03951.x

[15] Hammer H, Fox M, Keller J, Salvatore S, European H2-CH4-Breath Test Group, et al. European guideline on indications, performance, and clinical impact of hydrogen and methane breath tests in adult and pediatric patients: European Association for Gastroenterology, endoscopy and nutrition, European Society of Neurogastroenterology and Motility, and European Society for Paediatric Gastroenterology Hepatology and Nutrition consensus. United European Gastroenterology Journal. 2022;**10**(1):15-40. DOI: 10.1002/ueg2.12133

[16] Hammer J, Memaran N, Huber W, Hammer K. Development and validation of the paediatric carbohydrate perception questionnaire (pCPQ), an instrument for the assessment of carbohydrate-induced gastrointestinal symptoms in the paediatric population. Neurogastroenterology and Motility. 2020;**32**(12):e13934. DOI: 10.1111/nmo.13934

[17] Broekaert IJ, Borrelli O, Dolinsek J, Martin-de-Carpi J, et al. An ESPGHAN position paper on the use of breath testing in paediatric gastroenterology. Journal of Pediatric Gastroenterology and Nutrition. 2022;**74**(1):123-137. DOI: 10.1097/MPG.0000000000003245

[18] Nitescu M, Istratescu D, Preda C, et al. Role of an exclusion diet (reduced disaccharides, saturated fats, emulsifiers, red and ultra processed meats) in maintaining the remission of chronic inflammatory bowel disease in adults. Medicina. 2023;**59**:329. DOI: 10.3390/medicina59020329

[19] Johnson JM, Conforti FD. Fructose. In: Encyclopedia of Food Sciences and Nutrition. 2nd ed. 2003. p. 3472

[20] Efremowa I, Maslennikov R, Poluektova E, et al. Epidemiology of small intestinal bacterial overgrowth. World Journal of Gastroenterology. 2023;**14**(22):3400-3421. DOI: 10.3748/wjgv29.i22.3400

[21] Bushyhead D, Quigley EMM. Small intestinal bacterial overgrowth-pathophysiology and it's implications for definition and management. Gastroenterology. 2022;**163**:593-607

[22] Ghoshal U, Sachdeva S, Ghoshal U, et al. Asian-Pacific consensus on small intestinal bacterial overgrowth in gastrointestinal disorders: An initiative of the Indian neurogastroenterology and motility association. Indian Journal of Gastroenterology. 2022;**41**:483-507

[23] Skrzydło-Radomańska B, Cukrowska B. How to recognize and treat small intestinal bacterial overgrowth? Journal of Clinical Medicine. 2022;**11**:6017

[24] Andrei M, Gologan S, Stoicescu A, et al. Small intestinal bacterial overgrowth syndrome prevalence in Romanian patients with inflammatory bowel disease. Current Health Sciences Journal. 2016;**2**:151-156. DOI: 10.12865/ChSJ.42.02.06

[25] Rana S, Sharma S, Malik A, et al. Small intestinal bacterial overgrowth and orocecal transit time in patients of inflammatory bowel disease. Digestive Diseases and Sciences. 2013;**58**(9):2594-2598. DOI: 10.1007/s10620-013-2694-x

[26] Lee S, Falconer I, Madden T, Laidler P. Characteristics of oxygen concentration and the role of correction factor in real-time GI breath

test. BMJ Open Gastroenterology. 2021;**8**(1):e000640. DOI: 10.1136/bmjgast-2021-000640

[27] Lee J, Lee K, Chung Y, et al. Clinical significance of the glucose breath test in patients with inflammatory bowel disease. Journal of Gastroenterology and Hepatology. 2015;**30**:990-994

[28] Rezaie A, Buresi M, Lembo A, Lin H, et al. Hydrogen and methane-based breath testing in gastrointestinal disorders: The North American consensus. The American Journal of Gastroenterology. 2017;**112**(5):775-784. DOI: 10.1038/ajg.2017.46

[29] Nolan D, Han D, Lam J, et al. Genetic adult lactase persistence is associated with risk of Crohn's disease in the New Zealand population. BMC Research Notes. 2010;**3**(1):339

[30] Gu P, Patel D, Lakhoo K, et al. Breath test gas patterns in inflammatory bowel disease with concomitant irritable bowel syndrome-like syndromes: A controlled large-scale database linkage analysis. Digestive Diseases and Sciences. 2020;**65**:2388-2396. DOI: 10.1007/s10620-019-05967

[31] Wanzl J, Grohl K, Kafel A, et al. Impact of small intestinal bacterial overgrowth in patients with inflammatory bowel disease and other gastrointestinal disorders- a retrospective analysis in a tertiary single center and review of the literature. Journal of Clinical Medicine. 2023;**12**:935. DOI: 10.3399/jcm12030935

[32] Shah A, Morrison M, Burger D, et al. Systematic review with meta-analysis: The prevalence of small intestinal bacterial overgrowth in inflammatory bowel disease. Alimentary Pharmacology & Therapeutics. 2019;**49**(6):624-635. DOI: 10.1111/apt.15133

[33] Ricci Junior J, Chebli L, Ribeiro T, et al. Small intestinal bacterial overgrowth is associated with concurrent intestinal inflammation but not with systemic inflammation in Crohn's disease patients. Journal of Clinical Gastroenterology. 2018;**52**(6):530-536

[34] Wei J, Feng J, Chen L, et al. Small intestinal bacterial overgrowth is associated with clinical relapse in patients with quiescent Crohn's disease: A retrospective cohort study. The Annals of Translational Medicine. 2022;**10**(14):784. DOI: 10.21037/atm-22-3335

[35] Elguzebal N, Chamotto S, Molina E, et al. Lactase persistence, NOD2 status and Mycobacterium avium subsp. Paratuberculosis infection association to inflammatory bowel disease. Gut Pathogens. 2012;**4**(1):6

[36] Sanchez-Montez C, Ortiz V, Bastida G, et al. Small intestinal bacterial overgrowth in inactive Crohn's disease: Influence of thiopurine and biological treatment. World Journal of Gastroenterology. 2014;**20**(38):13999-14003. DOI: 10.3748/wjg.v20.i38.13999

[37] Nardone O, Manfellotto F, D'onofrio C, et al. Lactose intolerance assessed by analysis of genetic polymorphism, breath test and symptoms in patients with inflammatory bowel disease. Nutrients. 2021;**13**:1290. DOI: 10.3390/10.3390/nu13041290

[38] Kirschner B, De Favaro M, Jensen W. Lactose malabsorption in children and adolescent with inflammatory bowel disease. Gastroenterology. 1981;**81**:829-832

[39] Park R, Duncan R, Russel R. Hypolactasia and Crohn's disease. The American Journal of Gastroenterology. 1990;**85**:708-710

[40] Pfefferkorn D, Fitzgerald J, Croffie M, et al. Lactase deficiency: Not more common in pediatric patients with inflammatory bowel disease than in patients with chronic abdominal pain. Journal of Pediatric Gastroenterology and Nutrition. 2002;**35**(3):339-343

[41] Ratajczak A, Rychter A, Zawada A, et al. Lactose intolerance in patients with inflammatory bowel diseases and dietary management in prevention of osteoporosis. Nutrition. 2021;**82**:111043. DOI: 10.1016/j.nut.2020.111043

[42] Szilagyi A, Galiatsatos P, Xue X. Systematic review and meta-analysis of lactose digestion, its impact on intolerance and nutritional effects of dairy food restriction in inflammatory bowel diseases. Nutrition Journal. 2016;**15**:67. DOI: 10.1186/s12937-016-0183-8

[43] Mishkin S. Dairy sensitivity lactose malabsorption and elimination diets in inflammatory bowel diseases. The American Journal of Clinical Nutrition. 1997;**65**:564-567

[44] Tirpitz C, Kohn C, Steinkamp M, et al. Lactose intolerance in active Crohn's disease: Clinical value of duodenal lactase analysis. Journal of Clinical Gastroenterology. 2002;**34**(1):49-53. DOI: 10.1097/00004836-200201000-00009

[45] Wiecek S, Wos H, Radziewicz-Winnicki I, et al. Disaccharidase activity in children with inflammatory bowel disease. Turkish Journal of Gastroenterology. 2014;**25**(2):185-191

Chapter 4

Old and New Diagnostic Paths in Inflammatory Bowel Diseases

Giuseppe Leoncini, Simona Ronchetti, Rachele Del Sordo and Vincenzo Villanacci

Abstract

In the setting of the inflammatory bowel diseases, the role played by pathologists in the histological assessment of mucosal biopsy can be ideally divided into *four* steps. As a sequential proceeding, the histological evaluation has to deal with (1) the identification of the intestinal inflammation as consistent with ulcerative colitis or Crohn's disease, distinguishing them from their own mimickers; (2) the assessment of the inflammatory activity, thus highlighting their main descriptors, also including grade and distribution; (3) the evaluation of the histological features suggesting treatment response; (4) the histological detection of dysplasia and other complications in long-standing diseases. Requirements that should support the biopsy interpretation include (1) the thorough endoscopic data from the colonoscopy; (2) a comprehensive mucosal mapping; (3) a proper methodological approach to the mucosal specimens during the pre-analytical phase; (4) the methodological approach to the histological evaluation. In the last few years, efforts have been undertaken to identify novel histological markers of mucosal dysfunction in inflammatory bowel disease, which could help to identify novel markers of mucosal healing.

Keywords: inflammatory bowel disease, mucosal healing, scoring systems, dysplasia, glucocorticoid-induced leucine zipper (GILZ), mucins

1. Introduction

The term inflammatory bowel disease (IBD) refers to ulcerative colitis (UC) and Crohn's disease (CD), two chronic relapsing diseases involving the gastrointestinal (GI) tract and deeply affecting the patient's quality of life. Genetic, immunological and environmental factors have been advocated as pathogenetic contributors [1]. Recently, the weakness in the mucosal barrier has been proposed as an early causative co-agent in IBD onset [2]. The age of onset of UC and CD is variable and albeit adults are more commonly affected, both early and late onset can be seen in children and elderly respectively [3]. The main treatment goal in IBD is represented by the stable clinical remission, characterized by both symptomatic relief and mucosal healing. The medical treatment in IBD is mostly based on immunosuppression, through the administration of both anti-inflammatory and immunosuppressive drugs [4]. The suboptimal treatment and the long-lasting duration of the disease increase the risk of complications, including IBD-associated dysplasia and colorectal cancer (CRC). Both UC and CD are multifaceted diseases that need to be managed by multi-disciplinary teams [5].

2. Histological landmarks

2.1 Methodological approach

Before highlighting the main diagnostic clues in IBD, the methodological approach, encompassing both endoscopic and technical recommendations, should be considered. Notably, mucosal sampling should be performed on six gut segments, including the terminal ileum, cecum-ascending, transverse, descending, sigmoid colon and the rectum, collecting at least two pinch biopsies per each segment [6]. Then, mucosal specimens should be placed onto an acetate cellulose filter, in order to maximize the specimen's orientation [7, 8]. Since CD is known to not be limited to the gut, the clinical features can prompt to extend the endoscopic evaluation to the whole GI tract. In such cases, collecting two biopsies in both the esophagus and the duodenum, and five biopsies in the stomach, according to the Sydney scheme, is advisable [9]. The role played by processing and cutting should not be down-placed. Samples must be processed with the filter. A 90 degrees rotation of the filter-mucosal specimen must be performed before the embedding, in order to provide the proper trans-sectional orientation and to minimize manipulation artifacts. Relevant clinical, radiological and laboratory data should also be collected [8, 10]. Overall, the optimal recognition of the diagnostic clues of IBD, mostly the architectural abnormalities and basal plasmacytosis, also relies on methodology.

2.2 Ulcerative colitis

The UC can involve the colorectum with different extensions at the onset, ranging from proctitis and procto-sigmoiditis to left-sided disease and pancolitis. Disease progression across the colorectum can also occur. Unusual presentations include *rectal sparing and* the so-called *cecal patch*. Terminal ileum is spared by definition and, if involved, the suspicion of CD should be raised. However, mild inflammatory infiltration of terminal ileum can be observed mostly in pancolitis, and it is composed by lymphocytes, few plasma cells and neutrophils. Such finding is referred to as *backwash ileitis* and represents a reactive phenomenon that should not be misinterpreted as CD [11–13]. The histological features in UC can be grouped into *architectural* and *inflammatory abnormalities*. The *architectural abnormalities* refer to spatial alterations of glands, including glandular distortion, characterized by gland branching, fused or angulated glands and pseudo-villous mucosal surface. *Mucosal inflammation* is usually diffused in treatment-naïve UC, and it can be subdivided into *non-active inflammation* and *neutrophil-mediated (active) glandular injury* [8]. Non-active mucosal inflammation is composed by scattered lymphocytes, plasma cells and eosinophils into the lamina propria. Mucosal samples from active UC commonly exhibit abundant plasma cells infiltrate throughout the mucosal lining, and the involvement of the lower third (known as *basal plasmacytosis*) constitutes, along with the finding of architectural abnormalities, a diagnostic clue to distinguish UC from acute self-limiting colitis. Basal plasmacytosis is the strongest predictor of IBD, although differences in its segmental distribution were highlighted in UC and CD [14]. Few eosinophils are present in the healthy gut, with a slight predominance in the right colon and a gradient fading out towards the left colon. Increased eosinophils are detected in treatment-naïve UC, intermingled with plasma cells. The number, degranulation, clustering and intra-epithelial location of eosinophils have been related to a less responsiveness to corticosteroid drugs in UC patients [15].

Active inflammation is qualified by the presence of neutrophils into the lamina propria, also producing injuries on glands (cryptitis and crypt abscesses) and surface epithelium (erosions and ulcerations) [8]. Inflammatory pseudo-polyps result from severe mucosal damage in more aggressive diseases, representing the end-stage of the superficial epithelium injury. On the other hand, crypt lysis and atrophy, sometimes paired to *cryptolytic* granulomas, mark the end-stage of glandular injury [10, 16]. The active inflammation should be histologically graded and the three-tiered scheme, encompassing the mild, moderated and severe grades, is advisable (**Figure 1**) [17, 18].

2.3 Crohn's disease

The CD is characterized by trans-mural inflammation of the terminal ileum, but every segment can be involved in the GI tract. *Architectural changes* are commonly

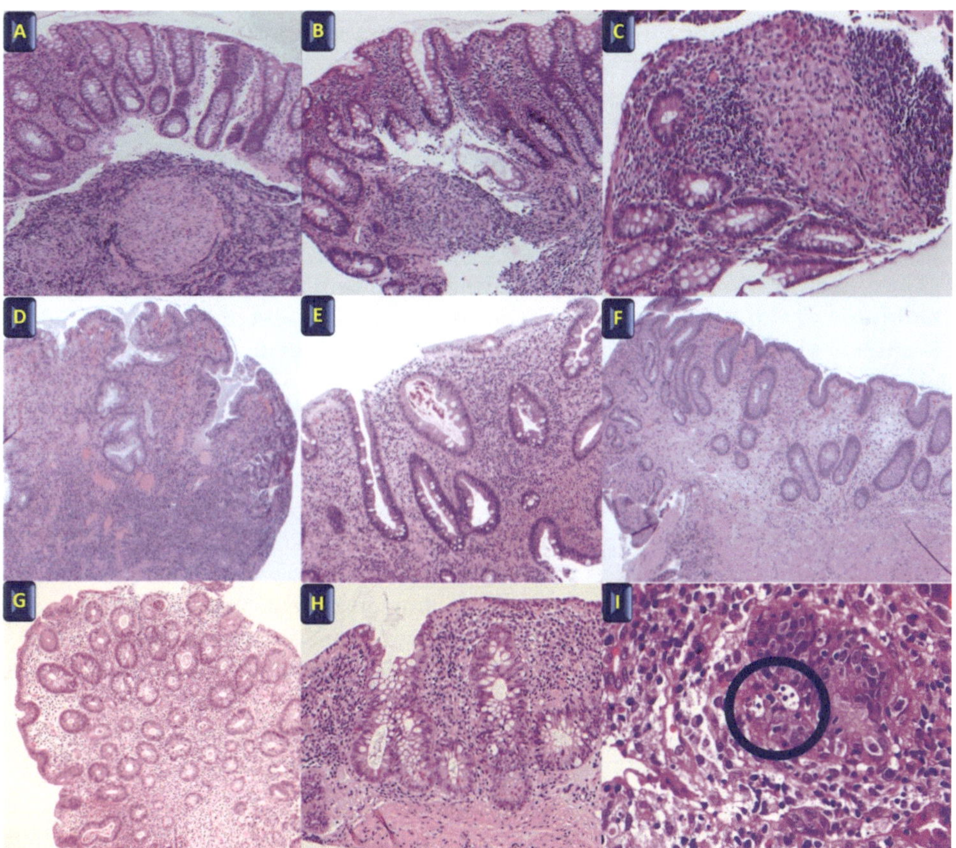

Figure 1.
A-B-C: Crohn's disease with the typical granulomas. H&E x 20. D-E-F: Ulcerative colitis D-E active H&E Dx10, E x 20, Fx10. G-H-I: Autoimmune colitis H&E Gx10, Hx20, Ix40 in the blu circle apoptotic body.

patchy, consisting in villous blunting in the small intestine, whilst glandular distortion is less prominent than that in UC and may involve few glands [8]. As in UC, *non-active inflammation* is composed by lymphocytes, plasma cells and eosinophils. The presence of neutrophils in the lamina propria qualifies the active inflammation and leads to epithelial injuries consisting in both glandular and surface lesions, even though gland cryptitis and abscesses are less extensive as compared to UC.

The discontinuous mucosal involvement represents another critical feature distinguishing CD from UC, resulting in patchy or segmental inflammation. Moreover, basal plasmacytosis is a less characteristic finding than in UC [19, 20]. The *early lesion* commonly consists in neutrophil infiltration of the superficial epithelium in the terminal ileum, leading to mucosal erosion and ulceration. Such erosive lesions can involve the mucosa overlying Peyer's patches, producing a peculiar histological feature called *aphtoid ulcer* [21]. The glandular injury leading to the mucus leakage in the lamina propria can evoke a local granulomatous reaction, promoting granuloma formation as in UC. However, such cryptolytic granulomas must be distinguished by typical epithelioid and non-caseating granulomas in CD.

Granulomas represent a characterizing feature in CD and are composed by discrete clusters of epithelioid histiocytes with intermingled T-lymphocytes. Granulomas in CD should be distinguished by cryptolytic granulomas, which are found close to injured glands. Conversely, CD granulomas are commonly detected in the lamina propria or at the edges of the inflammatory infiltration, and not in contact with glands. The sequential sectioning represents a basic requirement for the differential diagnosis [22]. In contrast with granulomatous enterocolitis caused by infective agents (e.g. Micobacterium sp., Yersinia sp), in which necrotizing granulomas can be detected, the CD is characterized by non-necrotizing granulomas (**Figure 1**) [23].

2.4 Typical findings in early and late onsets

The onset of IBD commonly involves the adult patients, but early and late onset in children and elderly respectively can be observed in a subset of patients [24–26]. IBD onset has been estimated to occur in about 25% of cases during childhood or adolescence [27].

In paediatric UC patients, the disease onset is characterized by the extensive colonic involvement in the majority of cases. Nonetheless, unusual presentations with patchy disease including caecal patch, and rectal sparing are not infrequent in children [28]. The early mucosal lesions are characterized by increased inflammatory infiltration into the lamina propria, including eosinophils and basal plasma cells [29]. However, architectural distortion and crypt atrophy pointing to the chronic nature of disease in the adult counterpart, are usually lacking in patients younger than 11 years [30]. Reactive changes in the terminal ileum, the so-called *backwash ileitis*, occur in approximately 20% of children presenting with pancolitis [31]. It consists of blunting of intestinal villi and mild neutrophil infiltration, often with patchy distribution, occasionally associated with crypt injury [32]. Detecting granulomas or pyloric metaplasia can support in distinguishing backwash ileitis from CD [33].

The CD onset usually involves the terminal ileum. The colonic involvement is seen in a lesser number of cases, often with rectal sparing. Isolated gastro-duodenal disease is observed in less than 5% of patients [34]. The early mucosal lesion consists in the patchy inflammatory infiltration of the lamina propria, with basal plasmacytosis, increased eosinophils and neutrophils. Non-caseating non-cryptolytic granulomas are more frequently observed in children than in adults [35]. The differential diagnosis mainly includes infectious colitis and food allergy. Moreover, the autoimmune enteropathy should be considered as a mimicker of IBD, mostly in patients suffering from IPEX syndrome (Immune dysregulation, polyendocrinopathy, enteropathy X-linked) and primary immunodeficiencies [36]. Gland atrophy, crypt hyperplasia and apoptotic bodies allow to discriminate autoimmune enteropathy from IBD (**Figure 1**). On the other hand, common variable immunodeficiency or severe combined immunodeficiency are characterized by reduced plasma cells into the inflammatory infiltrate [37].

Elderly patients are characterized by frequent co-morbidities, and a late onset of IBD commonly worsens their vulnerability, giving rise to daily challenges in the clinical management. There are not significant differences at histology in late onset UC, as compared to adult onset. However, elderly patients have a raised prevalence of non-IBD colitis that typically affects that subset of patients (e.g. the segmental colitis associated to diverticula - SCAD), which should be cautiously excluded. The CD can affect elderly patients, both resulting from a long-standing disease and as a late onset. Worth noting, terminal ileum has been reported to be less commonly involved in the late onset CD, the colonic involvement more frequently observed [38]. Moreover, a drug-induced injury should be considered in the differential diagnosis of Chron's ileitis in the elderly [39].

2.5 The mucosal healing: concept, practice and future perspectives

Medical treatment represents the first approach to IBD patients, aiming at earning symptomatic relief, as well as endoscopic and histological disappearing of mucosal inflammation. The general concept of *mucosal healing* (MH) emerged as the major treatment goal in IBD, predicting long-term remission. Moreover, MH correlates with a lower risk of IBD-associated dysplasia and CRC, being also related to lower rates of hospitalization and surgical procedures [40, 41]. The *endoscopic* MH is focused on the disappearing of inflammatory mucosal lesions at ileo-colonoscopy. However, there are no valid studies encompassing clinical-histological correlations on the topic [42]. Particularly, the histological features cannot be inferred by endoscopy, and the histological assessment of MH should be improved by pathologists, promoting simplified and highly reproducible scoring systems, as well as novel biomarkers.

At *histology*, neutrophil infiltration into the lamina propria is the most reliable histological marker of activity in IBD, also including neutrophil-mediated epithelial injuries. Hence, the absence of neutrophils and neutrophil-related mucosal injuries can be considered the most reproducible marker of histological MH. Furthermore, plasma cell infiltration is commonly seen in the lamina propria in IBD specimens and it is referred to as a marker of *chronic* inflammation [8]. However, the persistence of subtle plasma cell infiltration does not stand for active disease in treated patients, but conversely, it highlights the persistence of *chronic* inflammation [43]. Overall, the presence of plasma cells into mucosal biopsies from treated patients does not exclude the histological definition of MH, as long as neutrophils are absent.

During the last few years, efforts have been undertaken in order to identify markers that could support the histological definition of MH in IBD. The glucocorticoid-induced leucine zipper (GILZ) has been established to mediate glucocorticoid effects in immune cells, including T lymphocytes, B lymphocytes, macrophages and neutrophils [44–47]. Several *in vivo* models have been used to study the role that GILZ plays in inflammation, including IBD. Genetic ablation studies demonstrated the protective function of GILZ in IBD, due to the reduction of immune cell recruitment and activity in inflammation [48, 49]. Moreover, the administration of the recombinant GILZ protein has been proven to ameliorate symptoms of colitis in animal model studies, representing a novel pharmacological tool in IBD [50, 51]. Interestingly, GILZ has been recently established to play a secretory role in the gut, mostly involving goblet cells and enteroendocrine cells. Particularly, goblet cells showed a basal GILZ expression in normal colonic mucosa, whilst it was affected by active inflammation in IBD patients, with the expression reduced in active disease and restored in clinical remission [4]. Such GILZ dynamics correlated with neutrophil infiltration into the lamina propria, which represents the only reliable histological marker of activity in IBD. Importantly, the reduction or lack of GILZ in neutrophils exacerbates experimental colitis [46, 52]. Overall, GILZ expression can be considered a protective factor in the gut, its down-regulation marks the active phase of disease and its restoration strongly correlates with remission in IBD.

Furthermore, based on the recognition of the mucosal weakness as one of the major promoters of UC onset [2], colon-specific mucins (MUC) have been investigated in order to identify molecular traits of mucus barrier dysfunction. A novel signature involving MUC1, MUC4 and MUC5B derangements was found to characterize treatment-naïve UC patients. Moreover, the mucin expression profile was also found not to be restored in treated patients, who expressed the same types of mucin derangement. Notably, both relapsing and remitting patients showed commonalities in mucin expression profile with onset patients. Hence, evaluating the MUC1, MUC4 and MUC5B signatures should be integrated into the histological assessment of mucosal biopsies in treated UC patients. The assessment of gut mucin restoration should be integrated in the routine clinical practice as a functional descriptor of the histological MH. Worth-nothing, the proposed signature was also highlighted to represent an exploitable actionable target for specific MUC enhancers, opening novel treatment perspectives towards a synergistic approach, including immunosuppressive agents and mucin agonists [53].

3. The scoring systems in IBD

Several scoring systems have been proposed over time, aiming at grading disease activity and identifying histological MH. Such scoring systems considered and scored several histological parameters, including variations in inflammatory infiltrate, architectural abnormalities and epithelial injuries. However, validation studies are lacking for the most part of them, and their application into the routine clinical practice resulted to be complex, time-consuming and burdened by subjectivity [54, 55]. A *Simplified Histological MH Scheme (SHMHS)* has been recently proposed, being suitable for both CD and UC. It consisted in a two-steps approach, aiming at considering *neutrophil infiltration* as the major histological descriptor of activity, and *gut segments*. The SHMHS exhibited a high correlation rate with the endoscopic findings and resulted in simple, time-sparing and suitable for the clinical practice (**Table 1**) [43, 56, 57].

4. IBD-associated dysplasia and colorectal carcinoma

IBD is a well-recognized risk factor for CRC, with the risk of malignant transformation referred to be higher than that in a non-IBD population [58]. Increased

Features	Value	Score
Neutrophil infiltration into the lamina propria	Present	1
	Absent	0
Cryptitis and crypt abscesses	Present	1
	Absent	0
Erosion and ulcerations	Present	1
	Absent	0
Gut segments	*Value*	*Score*
Terminal Ileum (for CD only)	Quiescent	0
	Not involved	0
	Active	1
Right colon	Quiescent	0
	Not involved	0
	Active	1
Transverse colon	Quiescent	0
	Not involved	0
	Active	1
Descending colon	Quiescent	0
	Not involved	0
	Active	1
Sigmoid colon	Quiescent	0
	Not involved	0
	Active	1
Rectum	Quiescent	0
	Not involved	0
	Active	1

Table 1.
The simplified histological mucosal healing scheme (SHMHS).

risk of high-grade dysplasia and CRC in IBD patients with recurrent low-grade dysplasia [58]. Long-standing disease and ineffective treatments expose enterocytes to progressive oxidative stress, leading to mutagenic activity and carcinogenesis [59]. Particularly, p53 mutations mark the early phase of IBD-related carcinogenesis, in contrast with conventional CRC in which such mutations are found in the invasive phase [60]. Endoscopic surveillance plays a critical role in detecting early dysplastic lesions in IBD, monitoring clinical course and planning clinical management. The endoscopic features are listed into the scenic classification and encompassed both *visible* and *not visible* lesions. Visible lesions can present as polypoid, flat and depressed, as summarized in **Table 2**. Detecting dysplasia at histology represents the most reliable marker of malignant transformation in IBD patients, supporting clinical management and treatment planning. Worth noting, dysplasia that is found within the disease field, and referred to as *dysplasia associated lesion or mass (DALM),* should

Lesion type	Classification		Borders	Ulceration
Non-visible				
Visible	Polypoid	Pedunculated	Distinct	Present
		Sessile	Indistinct	Absent
	Non-polypoid	Superficial elevated		
		Flat		
		Depressed		

Table 2.
Scenic classification of endoscopic findings in IBD patients.

be distinguished from the so-called *adenoma-like mass (ALM)*, that arises outside, in bowel segments spared by inflammation, and that can be managed as sporadic adenomas. Unfortunately, detecting IBD-related dysplasia is burdened by high inter-observer variability, mostly in low grade and serrated lesions, and a *second look* is advisable to ensure the proper management of these patients [5].

5. The differential diagnosis in IBD

5.1 Drug-induced colitis

Drug-induced colitis (DIC) is an inflammatory condition in which the correlation with drugs administration is proven. DIC represents a prevalent cause of colitis in a specific population subset, mostly composed by elderly patients, often characterized by several vulnerabilities and co-morbidities [25]. Thus, the history of drug use should be clinically investigated, particularly in that subset of patients. Drugs and chemical compounds, including antibiotics, non-steroidal anti-inflammatory drugs (NSAIDs), laxatives, anticancer drugs and immunosuppressive agents, can induce cellular toxicity through allergic reactions and vascular insufficiency [61]. Watery diarrhea is the most complained symptom, whereas bloody discharge is seldom found and, if any, it is usually mild. Endoscopic findings can vary, ranging from unremarkable features to mucosal oedema and erythema with or without mucosal erosions. Worth noting, a normal-looking mucosa at endoscopy does not stand for healthy mucosa, thus a thorough mucosal sampling during ileo-colonoscopy is advisable [6].

The diagnosis of DIC needs thorough clinical-pathological correlations and the identification of one or more *inflammatory patterns* at histology (**Table 3**).

5.1.1 Pseudo-melanotic pattern

Lymphoid cells are commonly found in the gut mucosa, and their composition varies throughout the GI tract, including lymphocytes, granulocytes and histiocytes. Histiocytes are commonly found as scattered in the lamina propria and their *foamy-like* appearance is unusual in healthy mucosa. In the setting of DIC, the pseudo-melanotic pattern is characterized by the accumulation of histiocytes in the colonic mucosa, mostly in the upper third, but diffuse engulfment of the lamina propria can be seen in cases of long-term exposure to drugs. Pigment-laden histiocytes represent the most common finding, and can be found in loco-regional lymph nodes as well.

			Histological features	
DIC Patterns	**Lamina propria**	**Cell composition***	**Glandular features**	**Histological hallmarks**
Pseudo-melanotic	Hypocellular	Lymphocytes, plasma cells (few), histiocytes. Granulocytes uncommon.	Architectural sparing.# Epithelial injury uncommon.	Lipofuscin-laden histiocytes. Basal plasma cells absent.
Hyper-eosinophilic	Mild hyper-cellular	Eosinophils, lymphocytes, plasma cells (few), histiocytes. Neutrophils uncommon$	Architectural sparing.# Epithelial injury uncommon.	Eosinophil count (>60/10HPF). Basal plasma cells absent.
Acute inflammation	Hyper-cellular	Granulocytes (neutrophils and eosinophils), Lymphocytes, plasma cells (few), eosinophils (few).	Architectural sparing. #Epithelial injury common.	Acute inflammation with neutrophil-mediated epithelial injury. Basal plasma cells absent.
Ischemic	Hypocellular, Fibrotic	Lymphocytes, histiocytes, eosinophils (few). Neutrophils uncommon$	Architectural sparing. Atrophic changes	Atrophic glandular changes in fibrotic stroma. Basal plasma cells absent.
GVHD-like	Hypocellular	Lymphocytes, plasm cells eosinophils (few), histiocytes. Neutrophils uncommon$	Architectural sparing. Glandular hyperplasia	Raised apoptotic activity in glandular epithelium. Basal plasma cells absent.
Lymphocytic	Hypercellular	Lymphocytes, plasm cells eosinophils (few), histiocytes. Neutrophils uncommon$	Architectural sparing. Intra-epithelial T-lymphocytes	Diffuse intra-epithelial T-lymphocytes (>20/100 epithelial cells). Basal plasma cells absent.
Collagenous	Hypocellular Mild Hyper-cellular	Lymphocytes, plasm cells eosinophils (few), histiocytes.	Architectural sparing. Intra-epithelial T-lymphocytes (few)	Subepithelial collagenous band thickening (>10 μm). Basal plasma cells absent.

**Cell composition can vary according to the overlap with other DIC patterns;*
$unless an erosive process is associated, mostly in terminal ileum; and.
#referring to cryptitis and crypt abscesses, surface erosions and ulcerations.

Table 3.
Synopsis of the histological features in drug-induced colitis (DIC), according to the histological pattern.

Such lipofuscin-like pigment results from epithelial cell apoptosis with subsequent histiocytic phagocytosis occurring during contact laxative use (e.g. anthraquinone-containing drugs), even though it has also been described in NSAIDs abusers [61, 62]. Inflammatory infiltration is usually slightly increased into the lamina propria, but basal plasma cells are usually absent. The pseudo-melanotic pattern of injury can be also found to be associated with other patterns of DIC, particularly the focal active, hyper-eosinophilic and lymphocytic patterns. In those cases, the cellular composition varies in the lamina propria due to the enrichment of neutrophils, eosinophils and lymphocytes respectively. Glandular architecture is spared and there is not significant mucin depletion. Worth noting, the so-called "*melanosis coli*" has been linked to an increased risk of colonic dysplasia and CRC [63, 64].

5.1.2 Hyper-eosinophilic pattern

Colonic mucosa harbors eosinophils with a gradient decrease from the right to the left colon, and scattered eosinophils can be found in the small bowel as well. The main diagnostic clue in the hyper-eosinophilic pattern is detecting more than 60 eosinophils/10 high power fields [HPF] without peripheral hyper-eosinophilia [65]. The inflammatory infiltrate is slightly increased in the lamina propria, including lymphocytes and plasma cells, but basal plasmacytosis is usually absent. The hyper-eosinophilic pattern can occur alone or pair with other DIC patterns, including the pseudo-melanotic, lymphocytic and collagenous patterns [25]. In contrast with eosinophilic gastro-enteritis, eosinophilic colitis is a non-IgE-associated disease, with watery diarrhea as the most common clinical presentation [66]. Once parasitic infestations have been excluded, clinical-pathological correlations should be undertaken to distinguish drug-related colitis from gut diseases with an allergic etiology [65].

5.1.3 Acute inflammation pattern

This inflammatory pattern characterizes a broad and heterogeneous group of colitis, with different histological features, clinical presentation and causative agents. They range from focal acute colitis to pseudo-membranous and IBD-like colitis. Several drugs have been implicated, such as NSAIDs, antibiotics and laxatives [61].

In *focal active colitis,* the main histological clue is represented by neutrophil infiltration into the lamina propria, also promoting epithelial injuries (e.g. cryptitis, mucosal erosion). As focal active ileitis, it could give rise to the suspicion for CD onset. Worth noting, clues of chronic gut disease, including basal plasma cells and architectural distortion, are usually absent. Moreover, the presence of surface mucosal erosion along with a history of drugs use favor a drug-related etiology.

Pseudo-membranous colitis is a peculiar form of active colitis linked to Clostridium difficile infection, with both antibiotic therapy and older age representing the major risk factors. Pathologists should be confident with mucosal lesions in different evolutive phases. Particularly, the earliest type I lesion is rare and characterized by focal fibrin accumulation at the mucosal surface, oedematous lamina propria with scattered neutrophils and eosinophils. A small amount of weakly eosinophilic sub-epithelial exudate, surface erosion and focal cryptitis can be seen during this phase. In the type II lesion crypts are filled by eosinophils. The type III mucosal lesion represents the most severe mucosal injury, with diffuse coagulative necrosis, mucus accumulation, fibrin strands, cellular debris, neutrophils and eosinophils, constituting the typical *pseudo-membranes*. Type II and type III lesions should be distinguished from ischemic injury. Detecting collections of eosinophils in the crypt lumen aids the differential diagnosis, especially when a proper clinical-pathological correlation has been provided [67–69]. Some chemical compounds (e.g. gold salt) and drugs (e.g. NSAIDs, Micofenolate Mofetil) can produce an *IBD-like* pattern of injury consisting in some histological features frequently found in IBD, both in UC and CD. Active inflammation with surface mucosal erosions and ulcers paired to focal architectural abnormalities can be detected in the colonic mucosa, whilst the terminal ileum can present a cobblestone appearance resembling Crohn's ileitis [70, 71].

The acute inflammation pattern can be seen in combination with other DIC patterns of injury, most of all the hyper-eosinophilic and pseudo-melanotic patterns.

5.1.4 Ischemic pattern

Ischemic colitis can affect both young and elderly patients due to vascular and iatrogenic causes. Iatrogenic colitis with ischemic pattern is characterized by necrosis and inflammation, resulting from mucosal hypoxia. It results from non-occlusive etiology based on vasoconstrictive effect of drugs on small vessels [61, 72, 73]. Cocaine, amphetamines, diuretics and oral contraceptives have been implicated in this pathogenic mechanism [74, 75]. Glandular withering and coagulative necrosis characterize the mucosal injury at histology. Vascular congestion, haemorrhagic foci and capillary microthrombi may be also detected into the submucosal layer. Inflammatory infiltrate is usually mild, consisting in lymphocytes, plasma cells, histiocytes, and eosinophils, with a variable number of neutrophils. Basal plasma cells are usually absent. Architectural distortion is not a prominent finding, whereas small atrophic glands, lined by irregular cells with dark-stained nuclei, and variable degrees of fibrosis in the lamina propria can be found [76].

5.1.5 Apoptotic (GVHD-like) pattern

In transplant patients, the use of immunosuppressive agents (e.g. Micofenolate Mofetil) can give rise to adverse events including graft versus host disease (GVHD) and GVHD-like mucosal injuries. The same pattern of injury has been reported in patients who have not undergone transplants [77]. It refers to a peculiar mucosal damage caused by anti-inflammatory (e.g. anti- tumor necrosis factor (TNF) α, anti-interleukins/interleukin receptors) and anti-tumour drugs (immune checkpoint inhibitors, anti-CD20 and anti-endothelial growth factor). Diarrhea is the most frequently mentioned symptom and it is due to GI toxicity [78]. It should be noted that drug toxicity can cause other types of mucosal injury, including autoimmune enteropathy, acute and fulminant colitis, ischemic colitis, UC-like and CD-like inflammation. The *diagnostic clue* of the apoptotic pattern is represented by apoptotic epithelial cells at the base of the crypts [79–81].

5.2 Microscopic colitis

Microscopic colitis is a clinical term used to identify a clinical setting characterized by watery diarrhea and unremarkable endoscopic findings. Lymphocytic and collagenous colitis are the two histological findings in such cases, even though mixed forms can be seen. Microscopic colitis has several causative factors, including drugs (e.g. NSAIDs, PPI, ticlopidine) [82]. In lymphocytic colitis, the main *diagnostic clue* at histology is represented by diffuse infiltration of T (CD3+; CD8+)-lymphocytes (more than 20/100 epithelial cells) into the surface epithelium, the lamina propria is usually hypercellular, with neither architectural effacement nor basal plasma cells. On the other hand, collagenous colitis is qualified by thickening sub-epithelial collagen bundle (more than 10 μm), and inflammatory cells may present as either mildly or heavily increased into the lamina propria, but architectural abnormalities and basal plasma cells are usually unseen [83, 84]. Both lymphocytic and collagenous colitis can be found in combination with other DIC patterns of injury.

5.3 Infectious colitis

Infectious colitis is a self-limiting inflammatory disease involving the colonic mucosa, which may spontaneously resolve after time, most commonly a few weeks. Depending on the etiology, the onset of the disease is characterized by the increased number of inflammatory cells into the lamina propria, composed by lymphocytes, plasma cells, eosinophils and neutrophils. Epithelial injuries can be seen and could represent a prominent feature in the early phase of disease. Neither architectural distortion nor basal plasma cells are detected at histology, both representing a *diagnostic clue* for the differential diagnosis with active IBD. Moreover, some infectious species can promote histological features resembling IBD, making misdiagnoses possible. Particularly, colitis due to Campylobacter infection can be difficult to distinguish from active UC, whilst other microorganisms (e.g. Shigella species) can be associated with mucosal granulomatous reaction, suggesting to rule out CD [85]. Biopsy interpretation of infectious colitis relies on the absence of histological features pointing towards a chronic gut inflammation, particularly the absence of crypt distortion. Depending on the time of biopsy, we could have to deal with the resolving (late) phase of disease, presenting with different features at histology. The resolving phase of infectious colitis has a less cellular lamina propria, neutrophils are usually absent and, if any, they are scattered in the lamina propria and glandular damage is seldom found. The main *diagnostic clue* for the resolving phase is the recognition of increased apoptotic activity in the surface epithelium, which exhibits nuclear dust in a variable amount. Scattered intraepithelial lymphocytes (less than 20/100 epithelial cells) and regenerative hyperplastic changes in the surface and glandular epithelium can also be seen at histology [68, 86].

5.4 Segmental colitis associated to diverticulosis (SCAD)

The development of intestinal diverticula usually occurs asymptomatic. In symptomatic patients, medical treatment should be attempted, as significant morbidity may be associated with resection, especially in the elderly [87]. The SCAD refers to an inflammatory condition in which the sigmoid harboring diverticula shows different degrees of architectural distortion and inflammation, in a *segmental* fashion [88]. The inflammatory infiltrate is composed of lymphocytes, plasma cells, eosinophils and histiocytes. Basal plasma cells can be seen and neutrophilic infiltration promotes epithelial injuries [89]. Distinguishing SCAD from UC can be challenging on biopsy specimens, but the segmental distribution of inflammation represents the main *diagnostic clue*, since the rectum is spared by definition in SCAD, whereas it is involved in UC. Thus, the thorough mucosal sampling including biopsies from at least the rectum to the descending colon should not be omitted, in order to highlight the segmental nature of the inflammation in SCAD.

5.5 Ischemic colitis

Ischemic injuries can affect the large bowel following any of the following patterns: gangrenous colitis, haemorrhagic entero-colitis and ischemic colitis, the latter being due to subacute ischemic damage. It usually occurs in elderly patients mostly due to vascular causes. Hypoxia can produce two types of acute mucosal damage (gangrenous colitis and haemorrhagic entero-colitis) and a subacute injury (ischemic colitis) [90]. Young patients may also be affected due to drug abuse or systemic diseases (e.g. Behçet disease, systemic lupus erythematous) [91, 92]. It is characterized by mucosal injury, epithelial withering and coagulative epithelial necrosis at histology. In the submucosal layer vascular congestion, haemorrhagic foci and capillary microthrombi may be detected. Inflammation is usually mild and mainly composed by lymphocytes, histiocytes and granulocytes. Basal plasma cells are absent. Atrophic features of the glands, including clusters of small-sized glands with dark nuclei and condensed cytoplasm should not be misinterpreted as architectural distortion. Moreover, interstitial fibrosis can be found in the setting of chronic injury [76].

5.6 Radiation colitis

Radiation colitis is a treatment-related condition due to therapeutic irradiation of the abdomen, causing mucosal damage. The acute injury is represented by acute mucositis, whereas the chronic phase is characterized by progressive vascular damage and fibrosis [93]. Short-term lesions consist in mucosal inflammation and crypt abnormalities, epithelial reactive changes and apoptotic bodies are easily detectable in both the surface and glandular epithelium. Delayed injury can be subdivided into epithelial and stromal lesions, the former consisting in glandular alterations in size and shape, also exhibiting reactive epithelial changes that should not be misdiagnosed as dysplasia. Stromal alterations include fibrosis with atypical fibroblasts, and mild inflammation. Capillaries are usually dilated, with swollen endothelial cells and micro-thrombi. Small-sized arteries may show various degrees of lipid-laden macrophage into the intimal layer, wall hyalinization and fibrosis [94].

6. Conclusions

Managing patients suffering from IBD represents a daily challenge that must be addressed in the main clinical scenarios, consisting in 1) histological diagnosis; 2) evaluation of treatment response; 3) management of long-term complications, also including IBD-associated dysplasia and CRC. A multidisciplinary approach is advisable in every IBD clinical settings.

Acknowledgements

The present chapter is dedicated to Doctor Vincenzo Villanacci for the 10 years-long mentorship on gastrointestinal pathology, with gratitude.

Giuseppe Leoncini, MD.

Author details

Giuseppe Leoncini[1*], Simona Ronchetti[2], Rachele Del Sordo[3] and Vincenzo Villanacci[4]

1 Fondazione IRCCS Istituto Nazionale dei Tumori, Milan, Italy

2 Department of Medicine and Surgery, Section of Pharmacology, University of Perugia, Perugia, Italy

3 Department of Medicine and Surgery, Section of Anatomic Pathology and Histology, Medical School, University of Perugia, Perugia, Italy

4 Institute of Pathology ASST-Spedali Civili Brescia, Brescia, Italy

*Address all correspondence to: giuseppe.leoncini@istitutotumori.mi.it

References

[1] Kaplan GG. The global burden of IBD: From 2015 to 2025. Nature Reviews. Gastroenterology & Hepatology. 2015;**12**(12):720-727

[2] van der Post S, Jabbar KS, Birchenough G, Arike L, Akhtar N, Sjovall H, et al. Structural weakening of the colonic mucus barrier is an early event in ulcerative colitis pathogenesis. Gut. 2019;**68**(12):2142-2151

[3] Villanacci V, Reggiani-Bonetti L, Salviato T, Leoncini G, Cadei M, Albarello L, et al. A practical approach from the pathologists of the Italian group for the study of the gastrointestinal tract (GIPAD). Pathologica. 2021;**113**(1):39-53

[4] Leoncini G, Gentili M, Lusenti E, Caruso L, Calafa C, Migliorati G, et al. The novel role of glucocorticoid-induced leucine zipper as a marker of mucosal healing in inflammatory bowel diseases. Pharmacological Research. 2022;**182**:106353

[5] Leoncini G, Donato F, Reggiani-Bonetti L, Salviato T, Cadei M, Daperno M, et al. Diagnostic interobserver variability in Crohn's disease- and ulcerative colitis-associated dysplasia: A multicenter digital survey from the IG-IBD pathologists group. Techniques in Coloproctology. 2021;**25**(1):101-108

[6] Leoncini G, Bonzanini O, Bonfante FP, Polo S, Aimo G, Villanacci V. What to do when the large bowel looks like Normal. A retrospective analysis with clinical-pathological correlations. Digestive and Liver Disease. 2019;**51**:E151-E151

[7] Magro F, Langner C, Driessen A, Ensari A, Geboes K, Mantzaris GJ, et al. European consensus on the histopathology of inflammatory bowel disease. Journal of Crohn's & Colitis. 2013;**7**(10):827-851

[8] Villanacci V, Reggiani-Bonetti L, Caprioli F, Saragoni L, Salviato T, Mescoli C, et al. Histopathology of inflammatory bowel disease - position statement of the pathologists of the Italian Group for the Study of inflammatory bowel disease (IG-IBD) and Italian Group of Gastrointestinal Pathologists (GIPAD-SIAPEC). Digestive and Liver Disease. 2020;**52**(3):262-267

[9] Price AB. The Sydney system: Histological division. Journal of Gastroenterology and Hepatology. 1991;**6**(3):209-222

[10] Langner C, Magro F, Driessen A, Ensari A, Mantzaris GJ, Villanacci V, et al. The histopathological approach to inflammatory bowel disease: A practice guide. Virchows Archiv. 2014;**464**(5):511-527

[11] Joo M, Odze RD. Rectal sparing and skip lesions in ulcerative colitis: A comparative study of endoscopic and histologic findings in patients who underwent proctocolectomy. The American Journal of Surgical Pathology. 2010;**34**(5):689-696

[12] Odze R. Diagnostic problems and advances in inflammatory bowel disease. Modern Pathology. 2003;**16**(4):347-358

[13] Zimmer V, Emrich K. The cecal patch: A signature skip lesion in ulcerative colitis. Techniques in Coloproctology. 2020;**24**(2):213-214

[14] Villanacci V, Antonelli E, Reboldi G, Salemme M, Casella G, Bassotti G. Endoscopic biopsy samples

of naive "colitides" patients: Role of basal plasmacytosis. Journal of Crohn's & Colitis. 2014;**8**(11):1438-1443

[15] Leoncini G, Villanacci V, Marin MG, Crisafulli V, Cadei M, Antonelli E, et al. Colonic hypereosinophilia in ulcerative colitis may help to predict the failure of steroid therapy. Techniques in Coloproctology. 2018;**22**(12):941-946

[16] Gajendran M, Loganathan P, Jimenez G, Catinella AP, Ng N, Umapathy C, et al. A comprehensive review and update on ulcerative colitis(). Disease-a-Month. 2019;**65**(12):100851

[17] Villanacci V, Salemme M, Bassotti G, Antonelli E. Letter: Histological assessment of disease activity in ulcerative colitis--the problem of score evaluation and validation. Alimentary Pharmacology & Therapeutics. 2016;**43**(3):438-439

[18] Pai RK, Jairath V, Vande Casteele N, Rieder F, Parker CE, Lauwers GY. The emerging role of histologic disease activity assessment in ulcerative colitis. Gastrointestinal Endoscopy. 2018;**88**(6):887-898

[19] Torres J, Mehandru S, Colombel JF, Peyrin-Biroulet L. Crohn's disease. Lancet. 2017;**389**(10080):1741-1755

[20] Tanaka M, Saito H, Fukuda S, Sasaki Y, Munakata A, Kudo H. Simple mucosal biopsy criteria differentiating among Crohn disease, ulcerative colitis, and other forms of colitis: Measurement of validity. Scandinavian Journal of Gastroenterology. 2000;**35**(3):281-286

[21] Gullberg E, Soderholm JD. Peyer's patches and M cells as potential sites of the inflammatory onset in Crohn's disease. Annals of the New York Academy of Sciences. 2006;**1072**:218-232

[22] Qian Y, He W, Zheng CY, Xue JH, Fang JY, Chen XY, et al. Significance of granuloma and granulomatous lymphangitis in the differential diagnosis of Crohn's disease. Journal of Digestive Diseases. 2020;**21**(8):454-461

[23] Johnson CM, Hartman DJ, Ramos-Rivers C, Rao BB, Bhattacharya A, Regueiro M, et al. Epithelioid granulomas associate with increased severity and progression of Crohn's disease, based on 6-year follow-up. Clinical Gastroenterology and Hepatology. 2018;**16**(6):900-907 e1

[24] Sturm A, Maaser C, Mendall M, Karagiannis D, Karatzas P, Ipenburg N, et al. European Crohn's and Colitis organisation topical review on IBD in the elderly. Journal of Crohn's & Colitis. 2017;**11**(3):263-273

[25] Leoncini G, Reggiani-Bonetti L, Simoncelli G, Villanacci V. Histology of ibd and related colitides in the elderly. Minerva Gastroenterol (Torino). 2021. DOI: 10.23736/S2724-5985.21.02888-6

[26] Kuenzig ME, Fung SG, Marderfeld L, Mak JWY, Kaplan GG, Ng SC, et al. Twenty-first century trends in the global epidemiology of Pediatric-onset inflammatory bowel disease: Systematic review. Gastroenterology. 2022;**162**(4):1147-1159 e4

[27] Loftus EV Jr. Clinical epidemiology of inflammatory bowel disease: Incidence, prevalence, and environmental influences. Gastroenterology. 2004;**126**(6):1504-1517

[28] D'Haens G, Geboes K, Peeters M, Baert F, Ectors N, Rutgeerts P. Patchy cecal inflammation associated with distal ulcerative colitis: A prospective endoscopic study. The American Journal of Gastroenterology. 1997;**92**(8):1275-1279

[29] Kugathasan S, Judd RH, Hoffmann RG, Heikenen J, Telega G, Khan F, et al. Epidemiologic and clinical characteristics of children with newly diagnosed inflammatory bowel disease in Wisconsin: A statewide population-based study. The Journal of Pediatrics. 2003;**143**(4):525-531

[30] Glickman JN, Bousvaros A, Farraye FA, Zholudev A, Friedman S, Wang HH, et al. Pediatric patients with untreated ulcerative colitis may present initially with unusual morphologic findings. The American Journal of Surgical Pathology. 2004;**28**(2):190-197

[31] Levine A, Koletzko S, Turner D, Escher JC, Cucchiara S, de Ridder L, et al. ESPGHAN revised Porto criteria for the diagnosis of inflammatory bowel disease in children and adolescents. Journal of Pediatric Gastroenterology and Nutrition. 2014;**58**(6):795-806

[32] Yantiss RK, Odze RD. Diagnostic difficulties in inflammatory bowel disease pathology. Histopathology. 2006;**48**(2):116-132

[33] Koukoulis GK, Ke Y, Henley JD, Cummings OW. Detection of pyloric metaplasia may improve the biopsy diagnosis of Crohn's ileitis. Journal of Clinical Gastroenterology. 2002;**34**(2):141-143

[34] Lenaerts C, Roy CC, Vaillancourt M, Weber AM, Morin CL, Seidman E. High incidence of upper gastrointestinal tract involvement in children with Crohn disease. Pediatrics. 1989;**83**(5):777-781

[35] Rubio CA, Orrego A, Nesi G, Finkel Y. Frequency of epithelioid granulomas in colonoscopic biopsy specimens from paediatric and adult patients with Crohn's colitis. Journal of Clinical Pathology. 2007;**60**(11):1268-1272

[36] Daniels JA, Lederman HM, Maitra A, Montgomery EA. Gastrointestinal tract pathology in patients with common variable immunodeficiency (CVID): A clinicopathologic study and review. The American Journal of Surgical Pathology. 2007;**31**(12):1800-1812

[37] Russo P, Ruchelli ED, Piccoli DA. Pathology of Pediatric Gastrointestinal and Liver Disease. Second edition. Berlin: Springer; 2014

[38] Kedia S, Limdi JK, Ahuja V. Management of inflammatory bowel disease in older persons: Evolving paradigms. Intestinal Research. 2018;**16**(2):194-208

[39] Villanacci V, Bassotti G. Histopathological findings of extra-ileal manifestations at initial diagnosis of Crohn's disease-related ileitis. Virchows Archiv. 2017;**470**(5):595-596

[40] Mazzuoli S, Guglielmi FW, Antonelli E, Salemme M, Bassotti G, Villanacci V. Definition and evaluation of mucosal healing in clinical practice. Digestive and Liver Disease. 2013;**45**(12):969-977

[41] Antonelli E, Villanacci V, Bassotti G. Novel oral-targeted therapies for mucosal healing in ulcerative colitis. World Journal of Gastroenterology. 2018;**24**(47):5322-5330

[42] Sandborn WJ, Feagan BG, Hanauer SB, Lochs H, Lofberg R, Modigliani R, et al. A review of activity indices and efficacy endpoints for clinical trials of medical therapy in adults with Crohn's disease. Gastroenterology. 2002;**122**(2):512-530

[43] Villanacci V, Antonelli E, Lanzarotto F, Bozzola A, Cadei M, Bassotti G. Usefulness of different pathological scores to assess healing of the mucosa in inflammatory bowel

diseases: A real life study. Scientific Reports. 2017;**7**(1):6839

[44] Bruscoli S, Riccardi C, Ronchetti S. GILZ as a regulator of cell fate and inflammation. Cell. 2021;**11**(1)

[45] Hoppstadter J, Diesel B, Linnenberger R, Hachenthal N, Flamini S, Minet M, et al. Amplified host Defense by toll-like receptor-mediated downregulation of the glucocorticoid-induced leucine zipper (GILZ) in macrophages. Frontiers in Immunology. 2018;**9**:3111

[46] Ricci E, Ronchetti S, Gabrielli E, Pericolini E, Gentili M, Roselletti E, et al. GILZ restrains neutrophil activation by inhibiting the MAPK pathway. Journal of Leukocyte Biology. 2019;**105**(1):187-194

[47] Ricci E, Roselletti E, Gentili M, Sabbatini S, Perito S, Riccardi C, et al. Glucocorticoid-induced leucine zipper-mediated TLR2 downregulation accounts for reduced neutrophil activity following acute DEX treatment. Cell. 2021;**10**:(9)

[48] Bruscoli S, Sorcini D, Flamini S, Gagliardi A, Adamo F, Ronchetti S, et al. Glucocorticoid-induced leucine zipper inhibits interferon-gamma production in B cells and suppresses Colitis in mice. Frontiers in Immunology. 2018;**9**:1720

[49] Bereshchenko O, Coppo M, Bruscoli S, Biagioli M, Cimino M, Frammartino T, et al. GILZ promotes production of peripherally induced Treg cells and mediates the crosstalk between glucocorticoids and TGF-beta signaling. Cell Reports. 2014;**7**(2):464-475

[50] Ronchetti S, Gentili M, Ricci E, Migliorati G, Riccardi C. Glucocorticoid-induced leucine zipper as a druggable target in inflammatory bowel diseases. Inflammatory Bowel Diseases. 2020;**26**(7):1017-1025

[51] Gentili M, Hidalgo-Garcia L, Vezza T, Ricci E, Migliorati G, Rodriguez-Nogales A, et al. A recombinant glucocorticoid-induced leucine zipper protein ameliorates symptoms of dextran sulfate sodium-induced colitis by improving intestinal permeability. The FASEB Journal. 2021;**35**(11):e21950

[52] Ricci E, Ronchetti S, Pericolini E, Gabrielli E, Cari L, Gentili M, et al. Role of the glucocorticoid-induced leucine zipper gene in dexamethasone-induced inhibition of mouse neutrophil migration via control of annexin A1 expression. The FASEB Journal. 2017;**31**(7):3054-3065

[53] Leoncini G, Cari L, Ronchetti S, Donato F, Caruso L, Calafa C, et al. Mucin expression profiles in ulcerative Colitis: New insights on the histological mucosal healing. International Journal of Molecular Sciences. 2024;**25**:(3)

[54] Bryant RV, Winer S, Travis SP, Riddell RH. Systematic review: Histological remission in inflammatory bowel disease. Is 'complete' remission the new treatment paradigm? An IOIBD initiative. Journal of Crohn's & Colitis. 2014;**8**(12):1582-1597

[55] Mosli MH, Feagan BG, Zou G, Sandborn WJ, D'Haens G, Khanna R, et al. Reproducibility of histological assessments of disease activity in UC. Gut. 2015;**64**(11):1765-1773

[56] Caputo A, Parente P, Cadei M, Fassan M, Rispo A, Leoncini G, et al. Simplified histologic mucosal healing scheme (SHMHS) for inflammatory bowel disease: A nationwide multicenter study of performance and applicability. Techniques in Coloproctology. 2022;**26**(9):713-723

[57] Villanacci V, Del Sordo R, Parigi TL, Leoncini G, Bassotti G. Inflammatory bowel diseases: Does one histological

score fit all? Diagnostics (Basel). 2023;**13**:(12)

[58] de Jong ME, Kanne H, Nissen LHC, Drenth JPH, Derikx L, Hoentjen F. Increased risk of high-grade dysplasia and colorectal cancer in inflammatory bowel disease patients with recurrent low-grade dysplasia. Gastrointestinal Endoscopy. 2020;**91**(6):1334-1342 e1

[59] Zhang YZ, Li YY. Inflammatory bowel disease: Pathogenesis. World Journal of Gastroenterology. 2014;**20**(1):91-99

[60] Beaugerie L, Itzkowitz SH. Cancers complicating inflammatory bowel disease. The New England Journal of Medicine. 2015;**372**(15):1441-1452

[61] Geboes K, De Hertogh G, Ectors N. Drug-induced pathology in the large intestine. Diagnostic Histopathology. Springer. 2006;**12**:239-247

[62] Lee FD. Importance of apoptosis in the histopathology of drug related lesions in the large intestine. Journal of Clinical Pathology. 1993;**46**(2):118-122

[63] Li X, Zhou Y, Zhou S, Liu HR, Xu JM, Gao L, et al. Histopathology of melanosis coli and determination of its associated genes by comparative analysis of expression microarrays. Molecular Medicine Reports. 2015;**12**(4):5807-5815

[64] Puppa G, Colombari R. Brown colon (melanosis coli) harbouring pale tumors (adenocarcinoma and an adenomatous polyp). Journal of Gastrointestinal and Liver Diseases. 2009;**18**(4):509-511

[65] Casella G, Villanacci V, Fisogni S, Cambareri AR, Di Bella C, Corazzi N, et al. Colonic left-side increase of eosinophils: A clue to drug-related colitis in adults. Alimentary Pharmacology & Therapeutics. 2009;**29**(5):535-541

[66] Rothenberg ME. Eosinophilic gastrointestinal disorders (EGID). The Journal of Allergy and Clinical Immunology. 2004;**113**(1):11-28. quiz 29

[67] Price AB. Pathology of drug-associated gastrointestinal disease. British Journal of Clinical Pharmacology. 2003;**56**(5):477-482

[68] Villanacci V, Manenti S, Antonelli E, Chiudinelli M, Giuliano V, Bassotti G. Non-IBD colitides: Clinically useful histopathological clues. Revista Española de Enfermedades Digestivas. 2011;**103**(7):366-372

[69] Khor TS, Fujita H, Nagata K, Shimizu M, Lauwers GY. Biopsy interpretation of colonic biopsies when inflammatory bowel disease is excluded. Journal of Gastroenterology. 2012;**47**(3):226-248

[70] Dalle IJ, Maes BD, Geboes KP, Lemahieu W, Geboes K. Crohn's-like changes in the colon due to mycophenolate? Colorectal Disease. 2005;**7**(1):27-34

[71] Baert F, Hart J, Blackstone MO. A case of diclofenac-induced colitis with focal granulomatous change. The American Journal of Gastroenterology. 1995;**90**(10):1871-1873

[72] Feuerstadt P, Brandt LJ. Colon ischemia: Recent insights and advances. Current Gastroenterology Reports. 2010;**12**(5):383-390

[73] MacDonald PH. Ischaemic colitis. Best Practice & Research. Clinical Gastroenterology. 2002;**16**(1):51-61

[74] Beyer KL, Bickel JT, Butt JH. Ischemic colitis associated with dextroamphetamine use. Journal of Clinical Gastroenterology. 1991;**13**(2):198-201

[75] Tedesco FJ, Volpicelli NA, Moore FS. Estrogen- and progesterone-associated colitis: A disorder with clinical and endoscopic features mimicking Crohn's colitis. Gastrointestinal Endoscopy. 1982;**28**(4):247-249

[76] Habu Y, Tahashi Y, Kiyota K, Matsumura K, Hirota M, Inokuchi H, et al. Reevaluation of clinical features of ischemic colitis. Analysis of 68 consecutive cases diagnosed by early colonoscopy. Scandinavian Journal of Gastroenterology. 1996;**31**(9):881-886

[77] Villanacci V, Casella G, Bassotti G. The spectrum of drug-related colitides: Important entities, though frequently overlooked. Digestive and Liver Disease. 2011;**43**(7):523-528

[78] Papadimitriou JC, Cangro CB, Lustberg A, Khaled A, Nogueira J, Wiland A, et al. Histologic features of mycophenolate mofetil-related colitis: A graft-versus-host disease-like pattern. International Journal of Surgical Pathology. 2003;**11**(4):295-302

[79] Washington K, Jagasia M. Pathology of graft-versus-host disease in the gastrointestinal tract. Human Pathology. 2009;**40**(7):909-917

[80] Sale GE, Shulman HM, McDonald GB, Thomas ED. Gastrointestinal graft-versus-host disease in man. A clinicopathologic study of the rectal biopsy. The American Journal of Surgical Pathology. 1979;**3**(4):291-299

[81] Iqbal N, Salzman D, Lazenby AJ, Wilcox CM. Diagnosis of gastrointestinal graft-versus-host disease. The American Journal of Gastroenterology. 2000;**95**(11):3034-3038

[82] Fernández-Bañares F, Casanova MJ, Arguedas Y, Beltrán B, Busquets D, Fernández JM, et al. Current concepts on microscopic colitis: Evidence-based statements and recommendations of the Spanish microscopic Colitis group. Alimentary Pharmacology & Therapeutics. 2016;**43**(3):400-426

[83] Villanacci VSM, Microscopic colitis. In Colitis. A Practical Approach to colon Biopsy Interpretation, Geboes K.N.S., Leo M, Faa G editors, Ed. Springer: 2014; pp. 155-164

[84] Langner C, Aust D, Ensari A, Villanacci V, Becheanu G, Miehlke S, et al. Histology of microscopic colitis-review with a practical approach for pathologists. Histopathology. 2015;**66**(5):613-626

[85] Lamps LW. Infectious diseases of the lower gastrointestinal tract. Surgical Pathology Clinics. 2010;**3**(2):297-326

[86] Talbot I, Price A, Salto-Tellez M. Biopsy Pathology in Colorectal Disease. Second ed. London: CRC Press; 2006

[87] Sinclair A. Diverticular disease of the gastrointestinal tract. Primary Care. 2017;**44**(4):643

[88] Cuomo R, Barbara G, Pace F, Annese V, Bassotti G, Binda GA, et al. Italian consensus conference for colonic diverticulosis and diverticular disease. United European Gastroenterology Journal. 2014;**2**(5):413-442

[89] Tursi A, Inchingolo CD, Picchio M, Elisei W, Mangiola F, Gasbarrini G. Histopathology of segmental Colitis associated with diverticulosis resembles inflammatory bowel diseases. Journal of Clinical Gastroenterology. 2015;**49**(4):350-351

[90] Van Eyken P. F D, Gerosa C. Ischemic colitis. In: *Colitis. A Practical Approach to colon Biopsy Interpretation*. Geboes KNS,

Leo M, Faa G editors Ed. Springer: 2014. pp. 139-145

[91] Cai W, Zhu J, Hu D. Clinical features and risk factors for ischemic colitis in young and middle-aged patients. Acta Gastroenterologica Belgica. 2022;**85**(2):283-290

[92] Linder JD, Monkemuller KE, Raijman I, Johnson L, Lazenby AJ, Wilcox CM. Cocaine-associated ischemic colitis. Southern Medical Journal. 2000;**93**(9):909-913

[93] Willett CG, Ooi CJ, Zietman AL, Menon V, Goldberg S, Sands BE, et al. Acute and late toxicity of patients with inflammatory bowel disease undergoing irradiation for abdominal and pelvic neoplasms. International Journal of Radiation Oncology, Biology, Physics. 2000;**46**(4):995-998

[94] Leupin N, Curschmann J, Kranzbuhler H, Maurer CA, Laissue JA, Mazzucchelli L. Acute radiation colitis in patients treated with short-term preoperative radiotherapy for rectal cancer. The American Journal of Surgical Pathology. 2002;**26**(4):498-504

Chapter 5

Therapeutic Drug Monitoring in Inflammatory Bowel Disease

Anam Fahad, Somia Jamal Sheikh, Mishaal Munir, Asfand Yar Cheema, Muhammad Ali Khan, Hira Tahir, Rahimeen Rajpar, Ahmad Kasem, Sarayu Bhogoju, Hammad Qureshi and Syed Adeel Hassan

Abstract

Decades of cutting edge innovation in Inflammatory bowel disease (IBD) has yielded a diverse therapeutic armamentarium and warranted a shift in desired clinical endpoint (CE) from symptomatic management towards mucosal healing, histologic outcomes, serial biomarker trends and endoscopic remission. Despite these advancements, disease remission and therapeutic response rates remain suboptimal. This is due to failure to respond to therapy during the induction period (primary non-responder) or a subsequent loss of response (secondary non-responder). To address this area of unmet need, therapeutic drug monitoring (TDM) provides an opportunity to optimize dosing and therapeutic drug concentrations as per desired end clinical targets to improve response rates and offset aggressive disease complications. This further provides a platform for IBD therapeutic stratification based on patient, non-patient related factors and desired CE. In this chapter we aim to discuss a background regarding current TDM applications for various Food and Drug Administration (FDA)-approved IBD therapies and pinpoint deficiencies to enhance its smooth clinical implementation with a view to elucidating precision medicine as a novel therapeutic avenue in IBD.

Keywords: ulcerative colitis, Crohn's disease, antibodies, drug concentrations, drug monitoring, therapeutic drug monitoring, multi-utility, optimization

1. Introduction

Inflammatory bowel disease (IBD) is a chronic remitting and relapsing disorder comprised of Crohn's disease (CD), ulcerative colitis (UC) and indeterminate colitis [1]. Each disease subtype is classified based on location and extent of bowel wall involvement [1]. It is postulated that IBD-related intestinal inflammation is a consequence of aberrant immunological interaction between environmental, genetic and gut microbiome related factors [1]. In 1999, disease burden associated with IBD was estimated at 1.8 million (0.9%) in the American adult population [2]. However, as per recent extrapolations, the prevalence of IBD has substantially risen with as many as 3.1 million (1.3%) adults diagnosed with IBD [3]. As many as 70,000 new cases of

IBD are diagnosed each year further exacerbating the disease burden [4]. Likewise, the prevalence of IBD has risen 2 to 3 folds in the US veteran population [5].

The swift incorporation of immunomodulators, biologics and small molecules have revolutionized the management of IBD. Current Food and Drug Administration (FDA) approved therapies include thiopurines, tumor necrosis factor (TNF) inhibitors (infliximab, adalimumab, certolizumab pegol and golimumab), anti-integrins (vedolizumab, natalizumab), anti-interleukins (ustekinumab, risankizumab), janus-kinase inhibitors (upadacitinib, tofacitinib) and sphingosine 1-phosphate receptor modulators (ozanimod) [6]. The clinical heterogeneity of IBD is attributed to complex immuno-pathophysiological responses [7]. Improved understanding of underlying complex mechanisms and the availability of disease modifying therapeutic agents have warranted a shift in desired clinical outcomes from symptomatic management to well defined end points such as mucosal healing, histologic healing, serial biomarker trends and endoscopic remission with the goal of achieving durable deep remission (**Figure 1**) [8].

Despite a rapidly evolving therapeutic armamentarium, current literature suggests a perceived therapeutic ceiling attained with most therapeutic agents as evidenced by clinical remission rates leveling off at 40–50% [9]. Therapeutic response rates vary and remain suboptimal across drug classes. Only 50–60% of patients respond to therapy and obtain disease remission [10]. A further 50% of patients in remission eventually lose response to therapy [10]. This is attributable to absent clinical response post-induction (primary non-responder) or a loss of clinical response after initially attaining clinical response (secondary non-responder) [11]. Failure to therapy eventually results in the need for dose escalation or a switch in therapeutic class introducing higher odds of financial toxicity, recurrence of disease complications and hospitalizations [12]. To counter this unmet need, therapeutic drug monitoring (TDM) provides the opportunity to repurpose and optimize current modalities to directly improve patient outcomes.

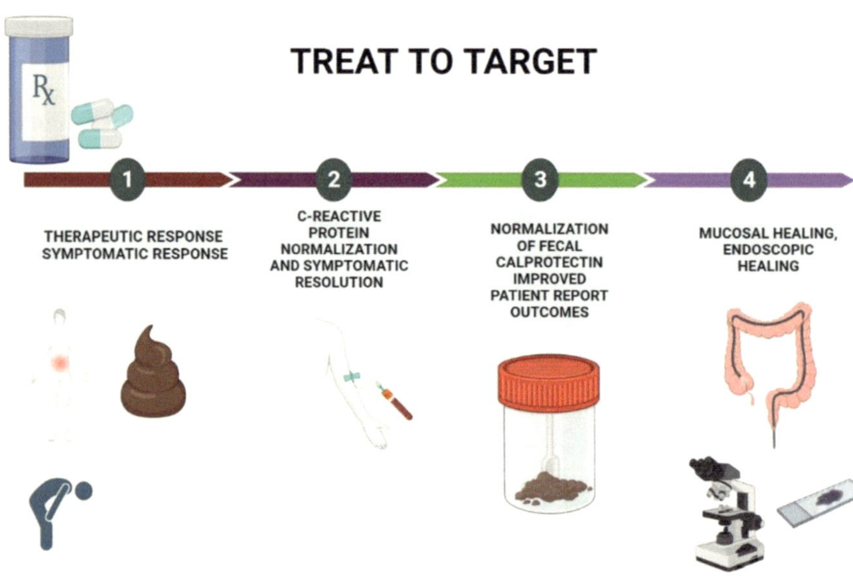
TREAT TO TARGET
Rx
1
2
3
4
THERAPEUTIC RESPONSE SYMPTOMATIC RESPONSE
C-REACTIVE PROTEIN NORMALIZATION AND SYMPTOMATIC RESOLUTION
NORMALIZATION OF FECAL CALPROTECTIN IMPROVED PATIENT REPORT OUTCOMES
MUCOSAL HEALING, ENDOSCOPIC HEALING

Figure 1.
Defined clinical end points desired as per increasing management timeline with treat to target approach. Created by BioRender.com.

TDM is a clinical decision making tool that quantifies serum drug concentration, active metabolites and anti-drug antibodies (ADA) to optimize treatment response [13]. Our current understanding of TDM is based on the results of multiple exposure-response studies that have delineated a positive association between higher drug/metabolite concentrations and desired clinical outcomes [13–16]. TDM allows incorporation of person-to-person variability in pharmacokinetic (PK) and pharmacodynamic (PD) factors that contribute to a loss of response (LOR) [13]. LOR tends to occur in the setting of low drug concentrations with/without ADA or an overall failure despite adequate drug levels [13]. These respective readouts guide dosing to achieve therapeutic concentrations/drug exposure associated with maximum therapeutic benefit. Exposure-response data are available for almost all therapies. However, most exposure-response studies have analyzed only anti-TNF therapy [13]. More recently, studies assessing the utility of TDM with anti-integrin and anti-interleukin therapy have come forth [17–20]. Innovation in antibody engineering have yielded newer biologics that are less immunogenic [21]. Therefore, the current rationale has also shifted from tackling immunogenicity to factors influencing drug exposure. Currently, almost all available IBD therapies have assays and TDM has become available for more modern therapies. Despite the implementation of TDM, there remains gaps that needs to be addressed to optimize its use in clinical practice. In this chapter we will review available evidence of TDM for various IBD therapeutic agents, utilization strategies and pinpoint deficiencies to improve current models of TDM [22].

2. Rationale for therapeutic drug monitoring

Our rationale for utilizing TDM is driven by data from multiple exposure-response studies suggesting strong association between clinical outcomes and serum drug concentrations [14]. Attaining optimal drug concentration is dependent upon several patient and drug related factors including but not limited to anti-drug antibodies, concomitant immunomodulator use, dose, disease phenotype, inflammatory burden, clinical end point, sample timing, sex, body mass and albumin levels [23, 24]. In a retrospective multicenter study, Juncadella et al. assessed biochemical, endoscopic and histological outcomes in 98 IBD patients treated with adalimumab who underwent TDM [25]. Findings from their study demonstrated that higher maintenance phase adalimumab serum concentrations >12 ug/mL were associated with both endoscopic and histologic remission [25]. Ungar et al. reported high rates of mucosal healing in patients with infliximab levels >6 ug/mL and adalimumab >8 ug/mL [26]. Similarly, Brandse et al. delineated a strong association between high serum drug concentrations in responders during induction with downstream desired clinical outcomes of endoscopic remission [27]. Likewise, studies have also showcased a poor association between low drug concentrations and clinical outcomes [14].

3. Mechanisms of drug failure

The availability of a myriad of therapeutic options can enforce premature cycling of drugs between different classes. This predisposes to premature drug discontinuation without effective dose optimization and incorrectly defining therapeutic failure. Particularly patients with refractory disease remain at risk of running short of therapeutic options with this approach. Therefore, it is imperative to better define and understand mechanisms underlying drug failure. This ensures maximum utilization of each drug class prior to a switch out of class.

3.1 Primary versus secondary non-response

Primary non-response (PNR) is defined as a lack of clinical improvement at the end of a defined induction period leading to discontinuation of therapy [28]. The incidence of PNR varies from 10 to 40% and is dependent upon the type of study design, definition of response and the type of therapeutic agent [29]. The time frames for assessment depends on the respective therapeutic class being utilized [28]. On the other hand, secondary non-response (SNR) is defined as worsening of symptoms indicating loss of response during the maintenance phase after having achieved clinical improvement during the induction period [28]. SNR is reported to occur in up to 50% of patients after 1 year of therapy [28].

The causative mechanisms for both are influenced by multiple factors including disease severity, disease phenotype, disease location, pharmacokinetics, pharmacodynamics, immunogenicity and dosing strategies [30]. Active smoking, low albumin, high inflammatory burden, presence of ADAs, high body mass index appears to lower response rates to TNFi (**Table 1**) [31]. Obesity also decreases time to LOR [32, 33]. It is postulated that obesity and low albumin increase drug clearance effectively reducing therapeutic drug concentrations [32, 33]. Patients with a history of prolonged disease duration (>2 years) are at a higher risk of developing PNR [34]. It is postulated that a longer disease duration is associated with a high burden of irreversible bowel damage impairing tissue integrity subsequently lowering response rates and patient outcomes [35]. Association between risk of PNR and disease location is well established in CD [36]. More specifically, small bowel and upper gastrointestinal CD is associated with a high risk of PNR [36]. Whereas colonic localization has shown improved response rates in patients undergoing TNFi therapy [36]. In summary, the underlying etiology remains poorly defined. However, the central theme remains inadequate drug concentrations during the induction or maintenance doses [28]. This is further backed by data from several recent studies delineating an association between inadequate serum drug concentrations and subsequent rates of therapeutic failure [14, 27, 37]. These risk factors need to be incorporated at the time of decision making to optimize risk based stratification for maximum drug utilization.

Factors	Effect
Weight	Increased drug clearance
Low Albumin	Increased drug clearance
>2 year disease history	Poor response rates due to effect on irreversible structural integrity and drug retention
Disease Type	Drug Clearance in UC > CD
Disease Activity	Drug clearance increased with higher inflammatory burden during active disease
Anti-Drug Antibodies	Increased Drug Clearance
Immunomodulator Use	Reduce Drug Clearance and formation of ADAs

Table 1.
Effect of risk factors on pharmacokinetics of anti-tumor necrosis factor therapy.

3.2 American gastroenterological consensus defined mechanisms

The AGA stratifies treatment failure based on drug trough and ADA levels in to three main causes including mechanistic failure, non-immune mediated pharmacokinetic failure and immune mediated pharmacokinetic failure [38]. As per the consensus determination, mechanistic failure also known as drug class failure should be suspected in patients not responding to therapy having attained optimal drug trough concentrations and undetectable ADA (**Figure 2**) [38]. These failures tend to present clinically as PNR early during the induction phase or later depicting a shift in underlying disease pathway as a mechanism to maintain ongoing inflammation [36]. This mechanistic escape eventually leads to the underlying disease process being driven by mediators not being targeted by that particular class of drug [38]. Therefore, the next best step in management for these patients represents a switch out of class to achieve response/remission [38].

The other 2 mechanisms pertain to pharmacokinetic (PK) failure and should be suspected in patients not responding to therapy in the setting of suboptimal drug concentrations [38]. They can be further sub-classified based on development of ADAs or non-immune drug clearance [38]. Non-immune mediated PK failure occurs in the setting of suboptimal drug concentrations and absent ADAs [38]. Non-immune failure can be mediated by sub-optimal dosing, low serum albumin, high body mass index, therapeutic non-compliance, high inflammatory burden associated drug clearance from reticuloendothelial system, gastrointestinal loss, drug wastage and varying drug distribution [14, 22, 38–40]. Patients presenting with non-immune failure can benefit from increasing drug dose or reducing dosing interval [41]. Immune mediated PK failure is suspected with high titers of ADAs and suboptimal drug concentrations [38]. The primary suspect for immune mediated failure are the drug neutralizing ADAs [38]. The most appropriate course of action in these cases is a switch within class [41].

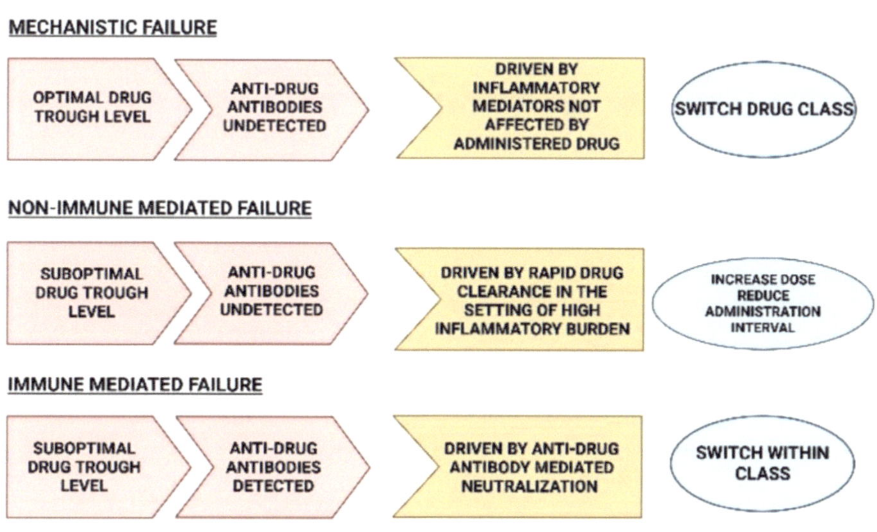

Figure 2.
Framework to identify mechanisms of treatment failure in inflammatory bowel disease as proposed by the American Gastroenterological Association consensus. Created by BioRender.com.

4. Available tools for therapeutic drug monitoring

Knowledge of current commercially available assays are critical to the implementation of TDM in the clinical setting. Current models quantify drug concentrations by measuring the trough level (TL) and anti-drug antibodies (ADA). TL is considered as the point of lowest concentration in relation to the already established drug threshold cut-offs at which efficacy is expected (**Figure 3**). [42, 43]. Current available assays allow monitoring of most IBD biologics including all TNFi, vedolizumab and ustekinumab. The 3 most commonly used assays are the radioimmunoassay (RIA), enzyme linked immunosorbent assay (ELSA) and homogenous mobility shift assay (HMSA) [44]. The most economical and commonly used assay in clinical practice is ELISA [44]. Each assay can be further subclassified on the basis of differential pre-analytical steps, antibody capture and antibody detection [44].

A natural question arises regarding the variation in performance of each assay. This led to multiple drug and anti-drug antibody comparative studies being conducted to assess individual performances [45–47]. Results from these studies helped establish the notion that good correlation exists among these assays for different drug concentration and anti-drug antibody titers [44–46]. Marini et al. evaluated infliximab concentration using four different commercially available ELISAs [48]. A strong correlation was noted with a coefficient of 0.89 for all tests [48]. When comparing inter-assay variability, ELISA, RIA, HMSA accurately detect serum drug concentrations ($r = 0.91–0.97$, $p < 0.0001$) [45]. Looking at individual assessment components, these assays are more reliable for producing specific, accurate and reproducible measures of drug TL [22]. The challenge remains in quantification of anti-drug antibodies due to variable readouts and requires careful derivation based on assay specific reference range [22]. Current guidelines recommend utilization of the same assay for checking both drug concentration and anti-drug antibodies in each patient [38].

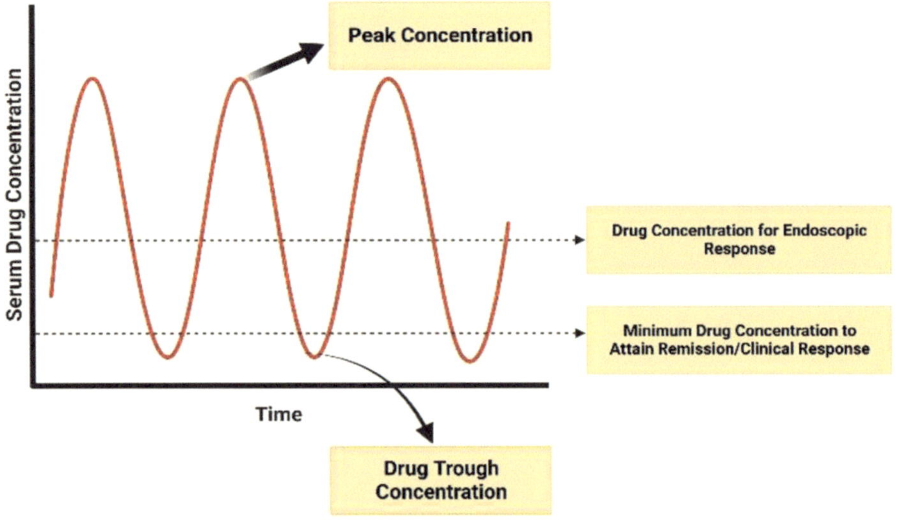

Figure 3.
Representation of terminology with respect to desired concentration targets.

5. Strategies for therapeutic drug monitoring

Prior to the availability of TDM, strategies involved in the management of therapeutic failure included empiric dose escalation, change within therapeutic class and switch outside therapeutic class. Even though this approach is thorough, it exposes the patients to trial with medications predisposing them to unnecessary adverse events. Additionally, these further delays initiating effective therapies and is associated with additional costs. While allowing for earlier implementation of effective therapies, TDM also provides a more personalized approach and is said to be more cost effective when compared to empiric therapy [49]. The utility of TDM varies based on clinical strategy. Current American Gastroenterological Association (AGA) guidelines recommend reactive TDM to guide dosing in patients with sub-optimal disease control [22]. Other possible clinical settings include proactive TDM during induction and maintenance phases, therapy de-escalation, drug holiday and toxicity prevention (**Figure 4**).

5.1 Reactive therapeutic drug monitoring

Reactive TDM evaluates serum drug concentrations and ADA to identify the mechanism of primary or secondary LOR in the setting of active IBD or intolerance to therapy [50]. It is considered standard of care in patients losing response to therapy [13, 38]. The most common causes of therapeutic failure with TNFi therapy is non-immune PK failure (51%) followed by mechanistic failure (30%) and ADA-mediated PK failure (19%) [22] An algorithmic approach helps stratify patients on the basis of TL and ADA [50]. With undetectable drug levels and no ADAs, decreasing drug interval or increasing the dose can benefit the patient [22]. At the same time adding an immunomodulator to reduce immunogenicity and increased drug levels should also be considered. A mechanistic failure should be suspected when drug levels are adequate with or without ADA [22]. This signifies an alternative inflammatory pathway driving disease and warrants a switch to a different class of drug. Finally, undetectable drug levels with the presence of ADAs suggest ADA mediated failure [22]. In this scenario, our next step in management depends on the titers of ADA. If ADA titers are low, addition of an immunomodulator can help re-gain response. However, if ADA titers are high, switching within drug class or to another class altogether represent possible options. A schematic of the decision making tree is presented in **Figure 5**.

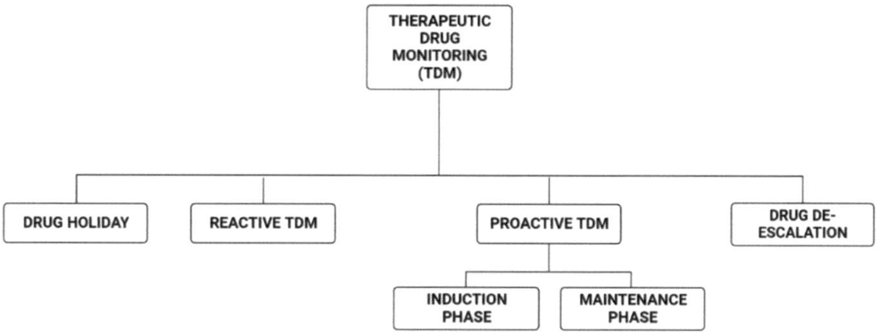

Figure 4.
Multiutility of TDM in inflammatory bowel disease. Created by Biorender.com.

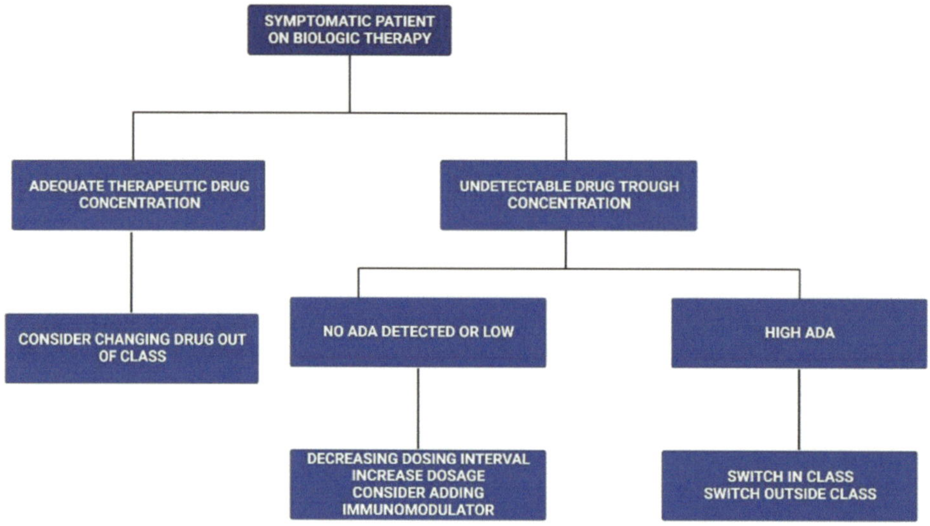

Figure 5.
Algorithmic approach to reactive TDM for biologic therapy.

In current literature, evidence regarding the utility of reactive TDM is stronger than that compared for proactive TDM. Additionally, most data pertains to the use of infliximab. Utilizing the algorithmic approach of reactive TDM helps better elucidate mechanisms associated with PNR. This provides an added benefit of minimizing inaccurate dose intensification in the setting of high ADAs [49]. In a retrospective study, Yanai et al. identified infliximab and adalimumab concentration cut offs at the time of SNR as an indicator of attaining downstream clinical benefit from a switch out of drug class or switching within class to another TNFi [40]. These cut offs are >3.8 ug/mL and > 4.5 ug/mL for infliximab and adalimumab respectively [40]. Roblin et al. utilized several infliximab decision algorithms as a model to extrapolate adalimumab pharmacokinetics [51]. At the time of SNR, adalimumab concentrations <4.9 ug/mL without ADA strongly predicted response to dose intensification in 67% of IBD patients [51]. Adalimumab concentrations >4.9 ug/mL were also associated with failure of 2 TNFi therapies [51]. Thus, adalimumab concentrations were also able to stratify patients that would require a switch out class [51].

In addition to rationalizing the treatment PNR and SNR, although controversial, we believe reactive TDM is non-inferior in terms of long term outcomes when compared with empiric therapy. In a retrospective observational study by Kelly et al., utilizing reactive TDM was associated with achieving a significantly higher post-adjustment clinical response and endoscopic remission [52]. Utilizing TDM was also found to lower rates of hospitalization [52]. In another study, Steenholdt et al. recruited 69 Danish CD patients receiving infliximab who had developed SNR [53]. They found similar rates of clinical response between patients with routine infliximab dose or TDM based intervention [53]. Interestingly, there was a 34% reduction in cost per patient in the TDM group [53]. The reduced cost of reactive TDM based dosing has also been well demonstrated in several other studies [54, 55].

5.2 Proactive therapeutic drug monitoring

Proactive TDM is defined as the assessment of drug trough concentrations and ADA at specific intervals to optimize dosing during induction, end of induction and maintenance phase [50]. The goal is to preemptively target optimal therapeutic range to prevent future LOR and disease flares [56]. This approach gained momentum due to data from exposure-outcome studies and post-hoc analysis of RCTs suggested an association between drug concentrations at specific time points and clinical outcomes when compared to reactive TDM and empiric dose escalation [25, 57–59]. The induction phase is a key period of interest due to high inflammatory burden, increased drug clearance and risk for inadequate drug exposure. Proactive TDM approach can help overcome these issues by early optimization of therapy [59].

In a study conducted by Papamichael et al., 101 UC patients were analyzed retrospectively [60]. The infliximab concentrations during induction was associated with short term mucosal healing [60]. In another multicenter study, outcomes were assessed for 102 IBD patients, patients undergoing proactive TDM had a greater drug persistence and reduced number of IBD related hospitalizations [61]. Papamichael et al. conducted another study in patients on adalimumab therapy where patients undergoing proactive TDM had a reduced risk of treatment failure compared to empiric therapy [22]. In the PAILOT study, a higher proportion of patients sustained steroid free remission and lowered biochemical markers with proactive adjustments of interval, dosing and drug trough concentrations when compared to reactive TDM [62]. In the landmark TAXIT trial, a lower frequency of undetectable drug levels, less antibody formation and lower disease flares were noted in the proactive TDM group [63]. The cost effectiveness of proactive TDM was recently assessed in a cost effective analysis of studies that utilized TDM with TNFi therapy [64]. Pooled assessment from

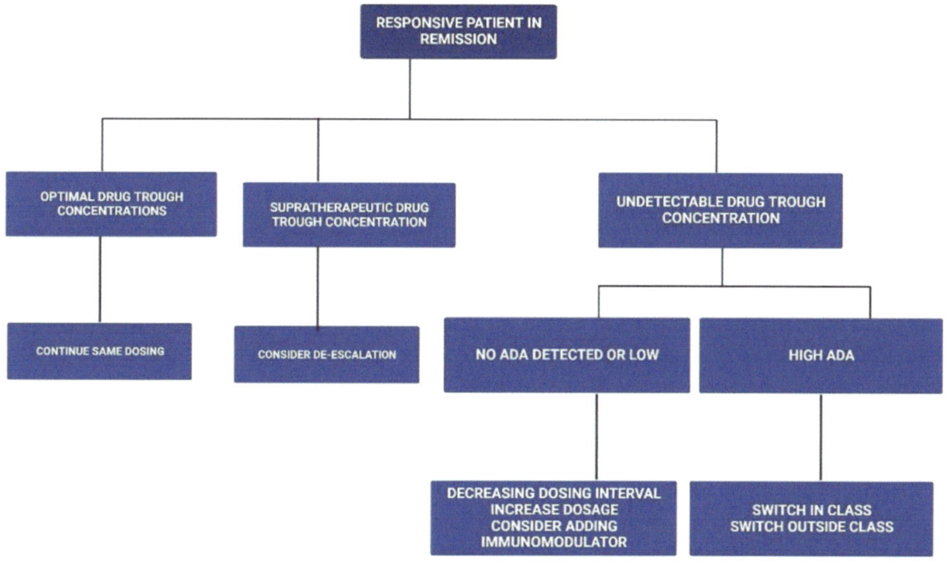

Figure 6.
Algorithmic approach to proactive TDM for biologic therapy.

4 modeling studies, 1 prospective observational study, 1 retrospective observational study, 1 NRCT and 1 RCT favor cost-effectiveness of proactive TDM [64]. Finally, a framework to approach proactive monitoring is provided in **Figure 6**.

5.3 Re-induction of therapy after drug holiday

A drug holiday is defined as a delay of ≥3 doses of biologic therapy [65]. Common reasons for a drug holiday include elective discontinuations due to surgery or infections, delayed insurance authorizations and stable remission [66]. In the setting of prior LOR to a biologic agent, re-induction with the same agent increases the risk of ADA formation and increases the odds of treatment failure. To prevent recurrence of treatment failure, the ACG endorses the use of proactive TDM to measure serum drug TL and ADAs after the first re-induction dose [67]. This also suggests that the greatest risk of infusion reactions is with the second re-induction dose [68]. In this scenario, TDM helps preempt PK failure due to possible inadequate drug exposure [67]. Currently, guidelines pertaining to the utility of proactive TDM for drug holidays are only established for infliximab [67].

Baert et al. evaluated 128 IBD patients who restarted infliximab therapy after a median discontinuation of 15 months [68]. Serum samples collected from prior trial of infliximab therapy were also analyzed for TL and ADAs [68]. Outcomes of this study included infusion reactions, TL, ADAs and response to treatment [68]. The absence of ADAs before second infusion and at re-initiation of therapy with immunomodulator use were associated with a clinical response [68]. Results from this study also suggested that early detection of antibodies to infliximab upon re-exposure resulted in higher infusion reactions [68]. Utilizing concomitant immunomodulator therapy to prevent development of ADAs and infusion reactions can help offset infusion reactions [68, 69].

5.4 De-escalate therapy

Commonly encountered in clinical practice, safety concerns warrant discontinuation of de-escalation from long term biologic and immunomodulatory combination therapy. In this setting, inappropriate de-escalation of biologic or immunomodulators can result in drop in biologic drug levels with a concomitant increase in immunogenicity. This increases risk of disease relapse and failure to maintain disease remission [69]. Proactive TDM can help measure both biologic and immunomodulator concentrations prior to treatment de-escalation. In the STORI trial, a low risk of relapse was seen in patients with low trough levels <2 mg/ul who discontinued infliximab after being on infliximab and thiopurine combination therapy [69]. Detectable infliximab trough levels at the time of immunomodulator discontinuation are also associated with long term response [70] Amiot et al. suggested de-escalation of infliximab therapy based on TDM rather than symptomatic and inflammatory burden stratification [71]. A real world cohort of 91 IBD patients in remission further showed that TDM is beneficial in delineating pharmacokinetic parameters helpful in the follow up of patients after biologic de-escalation [72]. As per the ACG consensus, dose de-escalation should be considered for infliximab or adalimumab for trough concentrations higher than 10–15 mg/ml [67].

6. Current guidelines for therapeutic drug monitoring

Despite the unavailability of large scale data, the use of TDM is supported by multiple medical societies globally [38, 56, 67]. In 2017, the AGA furnished guidelines to conditionally recommend the use of reactive TDM in adults with active IBD and receiving TNFi therapy [38]. These recommendations are limited to specific classes of TNF inhibitors and thiopurines. However, the use of proactive TDM is not currently recommended by guidelines [38]. Regardless, recent data suggests its active role in achieving favorable outcomes [61, 73]. Led by Cheifetz et al. the American College of Gastroenterology (ACG) published an expert consensus statement in 2021 [67]. In this report, the ACG encouraged the use of reactive TDM for all biologics [67]. They also recommended the use of proactive TDM for all TNFi therapy as well as under special circumstances such as drug holiday and therapy de-escalation [67]. Recommendations from ACG dug deeper in to utilizing TDM specific to disease subtype and activity [67]. In line with this, the ACG suggested the use of reactive TDM for UC relapse in patients with a history of moderate-severe UC [67]. However, no strong recommendations for CD were provided with the panel only suggesting reactive TDM in active CD [67].

7. Therapeutic drug monitoring for small drug molecules

7.1 Thiopurines

Initially developed for the treatment of acute lymphoblastic leukemia [74], thiopurines such azathioprine (AZA) and 6-mercaptopurine (6-MP) have proven to be quite effective in inducing steroid free remission in CD and UC [75–77]. In the current era, thiopurines are seldom used as monotherapy and are almost always used in combination with TNF inhibitors to enhance their therapeutic efficacy and minimize secondary LOR [78].

Thiopurines are pro-drugs that require extensive metabolism by multiple enzymes [79]. High inter-individual variability in its metabolism exists due to the requirement of specific target cell (leukocytes) and enzymatic activity [78]. AZA, 6-MP and thioguanines (TG) are converted into pharmacologically active 6-thioguanine nucleotides (6-TGN) namely 6-thioguanine monophosphate, 6-thioguanine diphosphate and 6-thioguanine triphosphate [78]. 6-TGN represents the pharmacologically active metabolites that eventually induce T-cell apoptosis [78]. Methylated metabolites are also of clinical interest as they are implicated in the development of thiopurine therapy associated toxicity [78]. Azathioprine undergoes direct conversion to 6-MP by removal of an imidazole group [78]. Subsequently, 6-MP gets metabolized to various metabolites via any one of three pathways [78]. The purine salvage pathways yields active 6-TGN metabolites by the enzyme hypoxanthine-guanine phosphoribosyl transferase [78]. Under the activity of thiopurine s-methyltransferase (TPMT), 6-methylmercaptopurine (6-MMP) are produced [78]. Incorporation of 6-TGN in to DNA and low TPMT activity have been associated with myelotoxicity [78]. High TPMT activity shunts the pathway towards increasing 6-MMP production, increasing drug toxicity and reducing downstream 6-TGN production resulting in reduced clinical efficacy [80]. Therefore, TPMT testing is important in determining if patients have reduced or absent TPMT activity. This ensures personalized dose reduction or selection alternative therapeutic agents. ACG recommends TPMT genotyping as it is a better representative of in vivo TPMT activity [67].

Dubinsky et al. proposed the utility of measuring metabolite concentrations (TGN and 6-MM) in erythrocytes along with pharmacogenomic profiling of TPMT genotype [81]. Despite the availability of tools to quantify these readouts, their role in the management of IBD are yet to be clarified [81]. A pooled analysis of 17 studies comprising of 2049 IBD patients established an association between 6-TGN metabolite levels and clinical remission [82]. A 3-fold increase in rate of clinical remission was noted in patients with 6-TGN levels >230–450 pmol/8 x 10^8 erythrocytes [83]. A cut off concentration of 397 pmol/8 x 10^8 erythrocytes have also been established for mucosal healing in CD [84]. Therapeutic non-compliance should be suspected if both 6-TGN and MMP are undetected [78]. Methodological and analytical assay limitations have limited further prospective assessments of thiopurine dose optimization in IBD [85, 86]. However, retrospective observational studies back the notion of introducing 6-TGN metabolite monitoring with clinical improvement noted in 6-TGN level driven dose optimization and significantly higher concentrations of 6-TGN in patients maintaining disease remission [87, 88]. Similarly, lower 6-TGN concentrations are also a feature of patients with active disease [88]. In addition to TPMT testing, thiopurine metabolite levels must also be quantified in a reactive setting and track toxicity [38]. As described above, cut off concentrations for thiopurine monotherapy have been well established. However, when used in combination with TNFi, 6-TGN cut off concentrations remain uncertain [38].

In the current therapeutic landscape, thiopurines are primarily used in conjunction with TNFi for sero-reversal of ADAs to reverse LOR, prevent LOR and immunogenicity to subsequent TNFi [89–91]. Their use has substantially declined due to the risk of malignancies [38]. More recently, studies have assessed the effect of proactive TDM on long term clinical outcomes. In a multicenter retrospective observational study, Barnes et al. assessed long term outcomes driven by thiopurine TDM interpreting 6-TGN and MMP metabolites [92]. In this largest retrospective cohort study of IBD patients receiving thiopurine, TDM was successful in optimizing dosage in 61.9% and enabled adherence to therapy [92] This approach of proactive TDM also improved clinical remission rates at the 1 year time point and accurately identified shunters that required addition of allopurinol to supplement therapeutic levels [92].

7.2 Methotrexate

Methotrexate is a folate antagonist (anti-metabolite) with antiproliferative, anti-inflammatory and immunosuppressive properties [93]. The efficacy of methotrexate monotherapy is well established in CD [94]. However, it failed to show any efficacy in UC [95]. The role of methotrexate is now limited to prevention of immunogenicity to TNFi. Adverse events associated with therapy include myelosuppression and hepatotoxicity [93]. A complete blood count and liver function test (LFT) must be ordered before and 1 month after initiation of therapy. Elevated LFTs warrant dose reduction whereas normal test results require maintenance of treatment with repeat testing every 3–4 months.

7.3 Sphingosine 1-phosphate receptor modulators

Ozanimod is a first in class sphingosine 1-phosphate (S1-p) receptor modulator that reduces circulating lymphocytes by blocking the egress from lymph nodes to inflamed tissue [96]. To date there are no exposure-response studies for this class of medication. The role of TDM remains to be further elucidated with data slowly emerging from efficacy and safety studies.

8. Therapeutic drug monitoring for biologics

8.1 Tumor necrosis factor inhibitors

Despite the availability of multiple agents in this drug class, our current understanding of the utility of TDM in TNFi is driven in majority by data from studies assessing infliximab or adalimumab. Very limited studies assessing exposure response relationships for certolizumab pegol and golimumab have been conducted to date. These studies have shown that higher drug concentrations are associated with better therapeutic outcomes in CD and UC respectively [97–99]. The role of TDM in infliximab have been thoroughly discussed in the strategies subsection.

With respect to proactive TDM in adalimumab, results from a multi-center retrospective study showed that the use of proactive monitoring performed superiorly than empiric dose escalation or reactive TDM by reducing rates of drug discontinuation, SNR, systemic adverse events or need for IBD related surgery [73]. In the PAILOT study, biologic naïve children who were responding to adalimumab therapy achieved higher rates of steroid-free clinical remission at week 72 when compared to reactive TDM [62]. From the perspective of reactive TDM, the EXTEND trial assessed the safety and efficacy of adalimumab in inducing and maintain mucosal healing [100]. It was concluded that patients undergoing reactive TDM were more likely to achieve mucosal healing [100].

8.2 Vedolizumab

Vedolizumab (VDZ) is a humanized IgG1 recombinant humanized monoclonal antibody approved for the treatment of moderate to severe CD and UC [101]. It prevents binding α4β7 integrins on naïve T and B lymphocytes and MADCAM-1 expressed on endothelial cells of the gastrointestinal tract and gut associated lymphoid tissue [101]. Hence, it tends to have a gut selective mode of action [101]. The therapeutic efficacy of VDZ was confirmed in the pivotal GEMINI I, II and III randomized control trials [102]. The recommended dose of VDZ is 300 mg with administrations at weeks 0, 2,6 during induction and every 8 weeks in the maintenance phase [102]. More recently, the efficacy and safety of subcutaneous administration of VDZ has been demonstrated in the VISIBLE trials [103]. Interestingly, the safety and efficacy profile of both standard IV and subcutaneous regimen are similar in both UC and CD for maintenance therapy [103].

When compared to TNFi, the correlation between clinical outcomes and VDZ concentration remain underpowered. During induction, initial association between VDZ concentrations and clinical efficacy were reported in the GEMINI trials [103]. Post-hoc analysis of GEMINI-I revealed a higher median CDZ trough levels during induction were associated with a significantly higher clinical remission rates at week 14 after induction therapy [104]. A weak association between week 6 VDZ trough concentrations and clinical outcomes with only a 22% remission rate in the higher quartile was noted in the GEMINI II and III trials [105]. To summarize, in UC patients, tough concentration increment from quartile 1 (≤ 17.1 ug/mL) to quartile 4 (> 35.7–140 ug/mL) was associated with a 31% increase in remission rate [106]. In CD patients, a 14% increase in remission rate was noted with a trough level increase from ≤16. ug/mL to 33.7 ug/mL [106, 107]. Studies have also helped demarcate VDZ trough cut-offs for mucosal healing and predicting the requirement for extended therapy.

A trough level < 18.5 ug/mL was associated with a need for extended therapy in the first 6 months [108]. Whereas a trough level > 18 ug/mL was associated with mucosal healing [108]. As per a recent expert consensus, VDZ drug level > 33–37 ug/mL at week 6 is recommended during induction.

With respect to exposure-response relationship in the maintenance phase, patients in the highest VDZ concentration quartile experienced a 20% increase in clinical remission at week 52 when compared with patients in the lowest quartile [56]. No relationship was delineated in patients receiving VDZ on a q4 basis [56]. Taken together, the utility of VDZ TDM is still under investigation. Data suggests a possible exposure-response relationship. However, clear thresholds/cut-offs have not been determined. Based on these findings, target VDZ concentrations of 33–37 ug/mL (week 6), 15–20 ug/mL at week 14 (end of induction) and 10–15 ug/mL during maintenance phase have been recommended to achieve improved clinical outcomes [104]. To date no studies comparing reactive and proactive approaches have been conducted. Therefore, there remains a need for a high quality data to help establish the role of TDM in utilizing VDZ.

8.3 Ustekinumab

Ustekinumab (UST) is an anti-interleukin agent which binds to the p-40 subunit of both interleukin-12 and interleukin-23 [109]. This prevents downstream interaction between these interleukins and their IL-12RB1 receptor reducing IL-12 and Il-23 mediated cell signaling [109]. Similar to VDZ, although limited, exposure-response relationship studies have shown an association between higher UST concentrations and improved outcomes [110–112]. UST concentrations >4.2 ug/mL during induction (week 8) were associated with a > 50% decrease in fecal calprotectin [112]. UST concentrations during maintenance have also been shown to be associated with biomarker reduction and endoscopic response [101, 112]. A UST trough level > 4.5 ug/mL was associated with an endoscopic response and lower mean c-reactive protein levels at week 26 [101]. A post-hoc analysis of the UNITI I/UNITI II trials revealed an association between clinical remission and week 8 UST trough concentration (>3.3 ug/mL, AUC =0.57) [113]. Patients with UST trough concentrations in the two highest quartiles in the UNITI I/II trials reported higher rates of clinical remission [113].

9. Challenges in current therapeutic drug monitoring models

Several limitations restrict the widespread implementation of TDM in IBD management. Current proactive assessment is limited to studies involving infliximab and adalimumab. The majority of these studies are retrospective in nature and increases the influence of selection bias. There is insufficient evidence to establish a trough level cut off for other biologics such as VDZ, UST, golimumab and certolizumab. Despite the availability of multiple commercially available assays, lack of standardization and guidance for interpreting results represents a major hurdle. Furthermore, there are no established cut-offs for ADA to differentiate between high titer versus low titer. Drug trough levels must not be considered absolute as they can be easily influenced by several factors such as smoking, body weight, inflammatory burden, disease severity and phase of therapy. Lack of standardized guidelines can also complicate the transition of TDM into clinical practice.

10. Conclusions

TDM is a versatile platform with the potential to revolutionize and personalize management of IBD. It involves measuring serum drug concentrations and anti-drug antibody levels to stratify mechanism of therapeutic failure and optimize management approach in the setting of loss of response. Current guidelines and evidence supports the use of reactive TDM. However, further methodologically accurate powered studies are needed to ascertain the proactive approach.

Acknowledgements

There are no acknowledgements to declare. No funding was received for this scientific work.

Conflict of interest

The authors declare no conflict of interest.

Author details

Anam Fahad[1], Somia Jamal Sheikh[2], Mishaal Munir[3], Asfand Yar Cheema[3], Muhammad Ali Khan[4], Hira Tahir[4], Rahimeen Rajpar[5], Ahmad Kasem[6], Sarayu Bhogoju[6], Hammad Qureshi[6] and Syed Adeel Hassan[6]*

1 Sahiwal Medical College, Sahiwal, Pakistan

2 Karachi Medical and Dental College, Karachi, Pakistan

3 Lahore Medical and Dental College, Lahore, Pakistan

4 Sheikh Khalifa Bin Zayed Al Nahyan Medical and Dental College, Lahore, Pakistan

5 Jinnah Sindh Medical University, Karachi, Pakistan

6 University of Kentucky, Lexington, USA

*Address all correspondence to: saha301@uky.edu

References

[1] Abraham C, Cho JH. Inflammatory bowel disease. The New England Journal of Medicine. 2009;**361**(21):2066-2078. DOI: 10.1056/NEJMra0804647

[2] Nguyen GC, Chong CA, Chong RY. National estimates of the burden of inflammatory bowel disease among racial and ethnic groups in the United States. Journal of Crohn's & Colitis. 2014;**8**(4):288-295. DOI: 10.1016/j.crohns.2013.09.001

[3] Kent KG. Prevalence of gastrointestinal disease in US military veterans under outpatient care at the veterans health administration. SAGE Open Medicine. 2021;**9**:20503121211049112. DOI: 10.1177/20503121211049112

[4] Colombel JF, Mahadevan U. Inflammatory bowel disease 2017: Innovations and changing paradigms. Gastroenterology. 2017;**152**(2):309-312. DOI: 10.1053/j.gastro.2016.12.004

[5] Hou JK, Kramer JR, Richardson P, Mei M, El-Serag HB. The incidence and prevalence of inflammatory bowel disease among U.S. veterans: A national cohort study. Inflammatory Bowel Diseases. 2013;**19**(5):1059-1064. DOI: 10.1097/MIB.0b013e31828028ca

[6] Zurba Y, Gros B, Shehab M. Exploring the Pipeline of Novel Therapies for Inflammatory Bowel Disease; State of the Art Review. Biomedicines. 2023;**11**(3):747. Published Mar 1 2023. DOI: 10.3390/biomedicines11030747

[7] Sudhakar P, Verstockt B, Cremer J, Verstockt S, Sabino J, Ferrante M, et al. Understanding the molecular drivers of disease heterogeneity in Crohn's disease using multi-omic data integration and network analysis. Inflammatory Bowel Diseases. 2021;**27**(6):870-886. DOI: 10.1093/ibd/izaa281

[8] Turner D, Ricciuto A, Lewis A, D'Amico F, Dhaliwal J, Griffiths AM, et al. STRIDE-II: An update on the selecting therapeutic targets in inflammatory bowel disease (STRIDE) initiative of the International Organization for the Study of IBD (IOIBD): Determining therapeutic goals for treat-to-target strategies in IBD. Gastroenterology. 2021;**160**(5):1570-1583. DOI: 10.1053/j.gastro.2020.12.031

[9] Raine T, Danese S. Breaking through the therapeutic ceiling: What will it take? Gastroenterology. 2022;**162**(5):1507-1511. DOI: 10.1053/j.gastro.2021.09.078

[10] Moss AC. Approach to treatment failure in inflammatory bowel disease. Gastroenterology Hepatology (N Y). 2022;**18**(6):360-363

[11] Vallejo-Yague E, Keystone EC, Kandhasamy S, Micheroli R, Finckh A, Burden AM. Primary and secondary non-response: in need of operational definitions in observational studies. Annals of the Rheumatic Diseases. 2021;**80**(8):961-964. DOI: 10.1136/annrheumdis-2021-220202

[12] Nguyen NH, Khera R, Dulai PS, Boland BS, Ohno-Machado L, Sandborn WJ, et al. National Estimates of financial hardship from medical bills and cost-related medication nonadherence in patients with inflammatory bowel diseases in the United States. Inflammatory Bowel Diseases. 2021;**27**(7):1068-1078. DOI: 10.1093/ibd/izaa266

[13] Papamichael K, Cheifetz AS, Melmed GY, Irving PM, Vande

Casteele N, Kozuch PL, et al. Appropriate therapeutic drug monitoring of biologic agents for patients with inflammatory bowel diseases. Clinical Gastroenterology and Hepatology. 2019;**17**(9):1655-68 e3. DOI: 10.1016/j.cgh.2019.03.037

[14] Kennedy NA, Heap GA, Green HD, Hamilton B, Bewshea C, Walker GJ, et al. Predictors of anti-TNF treatment failure in anti-TNF-naive patients with active luminal Crohn's disease: A prospective, multicentre, cohort study. The Lancet Gastroenterology & Hepatology. 2019;**4**(5):341-353. DOI: 10.1016/S2468-1253(19)30012-3

[15] Wilson A, Choi B, Sey M, Ponich T, Beaton M, Kim RB. High infliximab trough concentrations are associated with sustained histologic remission in inflammatory bowel disease: A prospective cohort study. BMC Gastroenterology. 2021;**21**(1):77. DOI: 10.1186/s12876-021-01650-7

[16] Ungar B, Engel T, Yablecovitch D, Lahat A, Lang A, Avidan B, et al. Prospective observational evaluation of time-dependency of Adalimumab immunogenicity and drug concentrations: The POETIC study. The American Journal of Gastroenterology. 2018;**113**(6):890-898. DOI: 10.1038/s41395-018-0073-0

[17] Walshe M, Borowski K, Battat R, Hudesman D, Wolf DC, Okada L, et al. Serum Ustekinumab concentrations are associated with remission in Crohn's disease defined by a serum-based endoscopic healing index. Crohns Colitis 360. 2021;**3**(3):otab032. DOI: 10.1093/crocol/otab032

[18] Yamashita N, Imai T, Kawahara M, Inatomi O, Andoh A. Low immunogenicity of vedolizumab determined by a simple drug-tolerant assay in patients with ulcerative colitis. Journal of Clinical Biochemistry and Nutrition. 2022;**70**(1):72-78. DOI: 10.3164/jcbn.21-98

[19] Nassar IO, Cheesbrough J, Quraishi MN, Sharma N. Proposed pathway for therapeutic drug monitoring and dose escalation of vedolizumab. Frontline Gastroenterology. 2022;**13**(5):430-435. DOI: 10.1136/flgastro-2021-102032

[20] Holmer AK, Battat R, Dulai PS, Vande Casteele N, Nguyen N, Jain A, et al. Biomarkers are associated with clinical and endoscopic outcomes with vedolizumab treatment in Crohn's disease. Therapeutic Advances in Gastroenterology. 2020;**13**:1756284820971214. DOI: 10.1177/1756284820971214

[21] Harding FA, Stickler MM, Razo J, DuBridge RB. The immunogenicity of humanized and fully human antibodies: Residual immunogenicity resides in the CDR regions. MAbs. 2010;**2**(3):256-265. DOI: 10.4161/mabs.2.3.11641

[22] Vande Casteele N, Herfarth H, Katz J, Falck-Ytter Y, Singh S. American Gastroenterological Association Institute technical review on the role of therapeutic drug monitoring in the management of inflammatory bowel diseases. Gastroenterology. 2017;**153**(3):835-57 e6. DOI: 10.1053/j.gastro.2017.07.031

[23] Irving PM, Gecse KB. Optimizing therapies using therapeutic drug monitoring: Current strategies and future perspectives. Gastroenterology. 2022;**162**(5):1512-1524. DOI: 10.1053/j.gastro.2022.02.014

[24] Hindryckx P, Novak G, Vande Casteele N, Laukens D, Parker C, Shackelton LM, et al. Review article: Dose optimisation of infliximab for acute

severe ulcerative colitis. Alimentary Pharmacology & Therapeutics. 2017;**45**(5):617-630. DOI: 10.1111/apt.13913

[25] Juncadella A, Papamichael K, Vaughn BP, Cheifetz AS. Maintenance Adalimumab concentrations are associated with biochemical, endoscopic, and histologic remission in inflammatory bowel disease. Digestive Diseases and Sciences. 2018;**63**(11):3067-3073. DOI: 10.1007/s10620-018-5202-5

[26] Ungar B, Levy I, Yavne Y, Yavzori M, Picard O, Fudim E, et al. Optimizing anti-TNF-alpha therapy: Serum levels of infliximab and Adalimumab are associated with mucosal healing in patients with inflammatory bowel diseases. Clinical Gastroenterology and Hepatology. 2016;**14**(4):550-7 e2. DOI: 10.1016/j.cgh.2015.10.025

[27] Brandse JF, Mathot RA, van der Kleij D, Rispens T, Ashruf Y, Jansen JM, et al. Pharmacokinetic features and presence of antidrug antibodies associate with response to infliximab induction therapy in patients with moderate to severe ulcerative colitis. Clinical Gastroenterology and Hepatology. 2016;**14**(2):251-8 e1-251-8 e2. DOI: 10.1016/j.cgh.2015.10.029

[28] Roda G, Jharap B, Neeraj N, Colombel JF. Loss of response to anti-TNFs: Definition, epidemiology, and management. Clinical and Translational Gastroenterology. 2016;7(1):e135. DOI: 10.1038/ctg.2015.63

[29] Ben-Horin S, Kopylov U, Chowers Y. Optimizing anti-TNF treatments in inflammatory bowel disease. Autoimmunity Reviews. 2014;**13**(1):24-30. DOI: 10.1016/j.autrev.2013.06.002

[30] Ding NS, Hart A, De Cruz P. Systematic review: Predicting and optimising response to anti-TNF therapy in Crohn's disease - algorithm for practical management. Alimentary Pharmacology & Therapeutics. 2016;**43**(1):30-51. DOI: 10.1111/apt.13445

[31] Arnott ID, McNeill G, Satsangi J. An analysis of factors influencing short-term and sustained response to infliximab treatment for Crohn's disease. Alimentary Pharmacology & Therapeutics. 2003;**17**(12):1451-1457. DOI: 10.1046/j.1365-2036.2003.01574.x

[32] Dotan I, Ron Y, Yanai H, Becker S, Fishman S, Yahav L, et al. Patient factors that increase infliximab clearance and shorten half-life in inflammatory bowel disease: A population pharmacokinetic study. Inflammatory Bowel Diseases. 2014;**20**(12):2247-2259. DOI: 10.1097/MIB.0000000000000212

[33] Harper JW, Sinanan MN, Zisman TL. Increased body mass index is associated with earlier time to loss of response to infliximab in patients with inflammatory bowel disease. Inflammatory Bowel Diseases. 2013;**19**(10):2118-2124. DOI: 10.1097/MIB.0b013e31829cf401

[34] Schreiber S, Colombel JF, Bloomfield R, Nikolaus S, Scholmerich J, Panes J, et al. Increased response and remission rates in short-duration Crohn's disease with subcutaneous certolizumab pegol: An analysis of PRECiSE 2 randomized maintenance trial data. The American Journal of Gastroenterology. 2010;**105**(7):1574-1582. DOI: 10.1038/ajg.2010.78

[35] Holmberg FEO, Pedersen J, Jorgensen P, Soendergaard C, Jensen KB, Nielsen OH. Intestinal barrier integrity and inflammatory bowel disease: Stem cell-based approaches to regenerate the barrier. Journal of Tissue Engineering and Regenerative Medicine. 2018;**12**(4):923-935. DOI: 10.1002/term.2506

[36] Vermeire S, Louis E, Carbonez A, Van Assche G, Noman M, Belaiche J, et al. Demographic and clinical parameters influencing the short-term outcome of anti-tumor necrosis factor (infliximab) treatment in Crohn's disease. The American Journal of Gastroenterology. 2002;**97**(9):2357-2363. DOI: 10.1111/j.1572-0241.2002.05991.x

[37] Brandse JF, Mould D, Smeekes O, Ashruf Y, Kuin S, Strik A, et al. A real-life population pharmacokinetic study reveals factors associated with clearance and immunogenicity of infliximab in inflammatory bowel disease. Inflammatory Bowel Diseases. 2017;**23**(4):650-660. DOI: 10.1097/MIB.0000000000001043

[38] Feuerstein JD, Nguyen GC, Kupfer SS, Falck-Ytter Y, Singh S. American Gastroenterological Association Institute clinical guidelines C. American Gastroenterological Association Institute guideline on therapeutic drug monitoring in inflammatory bowel disease. Gastroenterology. 2017;**153**(3):827-834. DOI: 10.1053/j.gastro.2017.07.032

[39] Paul S, Del Tedesco E, Marotte H, Rinaudo-Gaujous M, Moreau A, Phelip JM, et al. Therapeutic drug monitoring of infliximab and mucosal healing in inflammatory bowel disease: A prospective study. Inflammatory Bowel Diseases. 2013;**19**(12):2568-2576. DOI: 10.1097/MIB.0b013e3182a77b41

[40] Yanai H, Lichtenstein L, Assa A, Mazor Y, Weiss B, Levine A, et al. Levels of drug and antidrug antibodies are associated with outcome of interventions after loss of response to infliximab or adalimumab. Clinical Gastroenterology and Hepatology. 2015;**13**(3):522-30 e2. DOI: 10.1016/j.cgh.2014.07.029

[41] Fasanmade AA, Adedokun OJ, Ford J, Hernandez D, Johanns J, Hu C, et al. Population pharmacokinetic analysis of infliximab in patients with ulcerative colitis. European Journal of Clinical Pharmacology. 2009;**65**(12):1211-1228. DOI: 10.1007/s00228-009-0718-4

[42] Vaughn BP, Sandborn WJ, Cheifetz AS. Biologic concentration testing in inflammatory bowel disease. Inflammatory Bowel Diseases. 2015;**21**(6):1435-1442. DOI: 10.1097/MIB.0000000000000312

[43] Lobo ED, Hansen RJ, Balthasar JP. Antibody pharmacokinetics and pharmacodynamics. Journal of Pharmaceutical Sciences. 2004;**93**(11):2645-2668. DOI: 10.1002/jps.20178

[44] Vande CN. Assays for measurement of TNF antagonists in practice. Frontline Gastroenterology. 2017;**8**(4):236-242. DOI: 10.1136/flgastro-2016-100692

[45] Steenholdt C, Bendtzen K, Brynskov J, Thomsen OO, Ainsworth MA. Clinical implications of measuring drug and anti-drug antibodies by different assays when optimizing infliximab treatment failure in Crohn's disease: Post hoc analysis of a randomized controlled trial. The American Journal of Gastroenterology. 2014;**109**(7):1055-1064. DOI: 10.1038/ajg.2014.106

[46] Vande Casteele N, Buurman DJ, Sturkenboom MG, Kleibeuker JH, Vermeire S, Rispens T, et al. Detection of infliximab levels and anti-infliximab antibodies: A comparison of three different assays. Alimentary Pharmacology & Therapeutics. 2012;**36**(8):765-771. DOI: 10.1111/apt.12030

[47] Ruiz-Arguello B, del Agua AR, Torres N, Monasterio A, Martinez A, Nagore D. Comparison study of two

commercially available methods for the determination of infliximab, adalimumab, etanercept and anti-drug antibody levels. Clinical Chemistry and Laboratory Medicine. 2013;**51**(12):e287-e289. DOI: 10.1515/cclm-2013-0461

[48] Marini JC, Sendecki J, Cornillie F, Popp JW Jr, Black S, Blank M, et al. Comparisons of serum infliximab and antibodies-to-infliximab tests used in inflammatory bowel disease clinical trials of Remicade(R). The AAPS Journal. 2017;**19**(1):161-171. DOI: 10.1208/s12248-016-9981-3

[49] Ricciuto A, Dhaliwal J, Walters TD, Griffiths AM, Church PC. Clinical outcomes with therapeutic drug monitoring in inflammatory bowel disease: A systematic review with meta-analysis. Journal of Crohn's & Colitis. 2018;**12**(11):1302-1315. DOI: 10.1093/ecco-jcc/jjy109

[50] Vermeire S, Dreesen E, Papamichael K, Dubinsky MC. How, when, and for whom should we perform therapeutic drug monitoring? Clinical Gastroenterology and Hepatology. 2020;**18**(6):1291-1299. DOI: 10.1016/j.cgh.2019.09.041

[51] Roblin X, Rinaudo M, Del Tedesco E, Phelip JM, Genin C, Peyrin-Biroulet L, et al. Development of an algorithm incorporating pharmacokinetics of adalimumab in inflammatory bowel diseases. The American Journal of Gastroenterology. 2014;**109**(8):1250-1256. DOI: 10.1038/ajg.2014.146

[52] Kelly OB, Donnell SO, Stempak JM, Steinhart AH, Silverberg MS. Therapeutic drug monitoring to guide infliximab dose adjustment is associated with better endoscopic outcomes than clinical decision making alone in active inflammatory bowel disease. Inflammatory Bowel Diseases. 2017;**23**(7):1202-1209. DOI: 10.1097/MIB.0000000000001126

[53] Steenholdt C, Brynskov J, Thomsen OO, Munck LK, Fallingborg J, Christensen LA, et al. Individualised therapy is more cost-effective than dose intensification in patients with Crohn's disease who lose response to anti-TNF treatment: A randomised, controlled trial. Gut. 2014;**63**(6):919-927. DOI: 10.1136/gutjnl-2013-305279

[54] Guidi L, Pugliese D, Panici Tonucci T, Berrino A, Tolusso B, Basile M, et al. Therapeutic drug monitoring is more cost-effective than a clinically based approach in the Management of Loss of response to infliximab in inflammatory bowel disease: An observational multicentre study. Journal of Crohn's & Colitis. 2018;**12**(9):1079-1088. DOI: 10.1093/ecco-jcc/jjy076

[55] Velayos FS, Kahn JG, Sandborn WJ, Feagan BG. A test-based strategy is more cost effective than empiric dose escalation for patients with Crohn's disease who lose responsiveness to infliximab. Clinical Gastroenterology and Hepatology. 2013;**11**(6):654-666. DOI: 10.1016/j.cgh.2012.12.035

[56] Mitrev N, Vande Casteele N, Seow CH, Andrews JM, Connor SJ, Moore GT, et al. Review article: Consensus statements on therapeutic drug monitoring of anti-tumour necrosis factor therapy in inflammatory bowel diseases. Alimentary Pharmacology & Therapeutics. 2017;**46**(11-12):1037-1053. DOI: 10.1111/apt.14368

[57] Vaughn BP, Martinez-Vazquez M, Patwardhan VR, Moss AC, Sandborn WJ, Cheifetz AS. Proactive therapeutic concentration monitoring of infliximab

may improve outcomes for patients with inflammatory bowel disease: Results from a pilot observational study. Inflammatory Bowel Diseases. 2014;**20**(11):1996-2003. DOI: 10.1097/MIB.0000000000000156

[58] Roblin X, Marotte H, Rinaudo M, Del Tedesco E, Moreau A, Phelip JM, et al. Association between pharmacokinetics of adalimumab and mucosal healing in patients with inflammatory bowel diseases. Clinical Gastroenterology and Hepatology. 2014;**12**(1):80-4 e2. DOI: 10.1016/j.cgh.2013.07.010

[59] Sparrow MP, Papamichael K, Ward MG, Riviere P, Laharie D, Paul S, et al. Therapeutic drug monitoring of biologics during induction to prevent primary non-response. Journal of Crohn's & Colitis. 2020;**14**(4):542-556. DOI: 10.1093/ecco-jcc/jjz162

[60] Papamichael K, Van Stappen T, Vande Casteele N, Gils A, Billiet T, Tops S, et al. Infliximab concentration thresholds during induction therapy are associated with short-term mucosal healing in patients with ulcerative colitis. Clinical Gastroenterology and Hepatology. 2016;**14**(4):543-549. DOI: 10.1016/j.cgh.2015.11.014

[61] Papamichael K, Vajravelu RK, Vaughn BP, Osterman MT, Cheifetz AS. Proactive infliximab monitoring following reactive testing is associated with better clinical outcomes than reactive testing alone in patients with inflammatory bowel disease. Journal of Crohn's & Colitis. 2018;**12**(7):804-810. DOI: 10.1093/ecco-jcc/jjy039

[62] Assa A, Matar M, Turner D, Broide E, Weiss B, Ledder O, et al. Proactive monitoring of Adalimumab trough concentration associated with increased clinical remission in children with Crohn's disease compared with reactive monitoring. Gastroenterology. 2019;**157**(4):985-96 e2. DOI: 10.1053/j.gastro.2019.06.003

[63] Vande Casteele N, Ferrante M, Van Assche G, Ballet V, Compernolle G, Van Steen K, et al. Trough concentrations of infliximab guide dosing for patients with inflammatory bowel disease. Gastroenterology. 2015;**148**(7):1320-9 e3. DOI: 10.1053/j.gastro.2015.02.031

[64] Marquez-Megias S, Nalda-Molina R, Sanz-Valero J, et al. Cost-Effectiveness of Therapeutic Drug Monitoring of Anti-TNF Therapy in Inflammatory Bowel Disease: A Systematic Review. Pharmaceutics. 2022;**14**(5):1009. Published May 7 2022. DOI: 10.3390/pharmaceutics14051009

[65] Melmed GY, Irving PM, Jones J, Kaplan GG, Kozuch PL, Velayos FS, et al. Appropriateness of testing for anti-tumor necrosis factor agent and antibody concentrations, and interpretation of results. Clinical Gastroenterology and Hepatology. 2016;**14**(9):1302-1309. DOI: 10.1016/j.cgh.2016.05.010

[66] Rubin DT. Restarting biologic agents after a drug holiday. Gastroenterology Hepatology (N Y). 2019;**15**(11, 5):612

[67] Cheifetz AS, Abreu MT, Afif W, Cross RK, Dubinsky MC, Loftus EV Jr, et al. A comprehensive literature review and expert consensus statement on therapeutic drug monitoring of biologics in inflammatory bowel disease. The American Journal of Gastroenterology. 2021;**116**(10):2014-2025. DOI: 10.14309/ajg.0000000000001396

[68] Baert F, Drobne D, Gils A, Vande Casteele N, Hauenstein S, Singh S, et al. Early trough levels and antibodies to infliximab predict safety and

success of reinitiation of infliximab therapy. Clinical Gastroenterology and Hepatology 2014;12(9):1474-1481 e2; quiz e91. DOI: 10.1016/j.cgh.2014.01.033.

[69] Louis E, Mary JY, Vernier-Massouille G, Grimaud JC, Bouhnik Y, Laharie D, et al. Maintenance of remission among patients with Crohn's disease on antimetabolite therapy after infliximab therapy is stopped. Gastroenterology 2012;142(1):63-70 e5; quiz e31. DOI: 10.1053/j.gastro.2011.09.034.

[70] Drobne D, Bossuyt P, Breynaert C, Cattaert T, Vande Casteele N, Compernolle G, et al. Withdrawal of immunomodulators after co-treatment does not reduce trough level of infliximab in patients with Crohn's disease. Clinical Gastroenterology and Hepatology. 2015;**13**(3):514-21 e4. DOI: 10.1016/j.cgh.2014.07.027

[71] Amiot A, Hulin A, Belhassan M, Andre C, Gagniere C, Le Baleur Y, et al. Therapeutic drug monitoring is predictive of loss of response after de-escalation of infliximab therapy in patients with inflammatory bowel disease in clinical remission. Clinics and Research in Hepatology and Gastroenterology. 2016;**40**(1):90-98. DOI: 10.1016/j.clinre.2015.05.019

[72] Petitcollin A, Brochard C, Siproudhis L, Tron C, Verdier MC, Lemaitre F, et al. Pharmacokinetic parameters of infliximab influence the rate of relapse after De-escalation in adults with inflammatory bowel diseases. Clinical Pharmacology and Therapeutics. 2019;**106**(3):605-615. DOI: 10.1002/cpt.1429

[73] Papamichael K, Juncadella A, Wong D, Rakowsky S, Sattler LA, Campbell JP, et al. Proactive therapeutic drug monitoring of Adalimumab is associated with better long-term outcomes compared with standard of Care in Patients with Inflammatory Bowel Disease. Journal of Crohn's & Colitis. 2019;**13**(8):976-981. DOI: 10.1093/ecco-jcc/jjz018

[74] Elion GB. The purine path to chemotherapy. Science. 1989;**244**(4900): 41-47. DOI: 10.1126/science.2649979

[75] Ardizzone S, Bollani S, Manzionna G, Imbesi V, Colombo E, Bianchi PG. Comparison between methotrexate and azathioprine in the treatment of chronic active Crohn's disease: A randomised, investigator-blind study. Digestive and Liver Disease. 2003;**35**(9):619-627. DOI: 10.1016/s1590-8658(03)00372-4

[76] Candy S, Wright J, Gerber M, Adams G, Gerig M, Goodman R. A controlled double blind study of azathioprine in the management of Crohn's disease. Gut. 1995;**37**(5):674-678. DOI: 10.1136/gut.37.5.674

[77] Israeli E, Goldin E, Fishman S, Konikoff F, Lavy A, Chowers Y, et al. Oral administration of non-absorbable delayed release 6-mercaptopurine is locally active in the gut, exerts a systemic immune effect and alleviates Crohn's disease with low rate of side effects: Results of double blind phase II clinical trial. Clinical and Experimental Immunology. 2015;**181**(2):362-372. DOI: 10.1111/cei.12640

[78] Simsek M, Meijer B, Mulder CJJ, van Bodegraven AA, de Boer NKH. Analytical pitfalls of therapeutic drug monitoring of Thiopurines in patients with inflammatory bowel disease. Therapeutic Drug Monitoring. 2017;**39**(6):584-588. DOI: 10.1097/FTD.0000000000000455

[79] Quemeneur L, Gerland LM, Flacher M, Ffrench M, Revillard JP, Genestier L. Differential control of

cell cycle, proliferation, and survival of primary T lymphocytes by purine and pyrimidine nucleotides. Journal of Immunology. 2003;**170**(10):4986-4995. DOI: 10.4049/jimmunol.170.10.4986

[80] Derijks LJ, Gilissen LP, Hooymans PM, Hommes DW. Review article: Thiopurines in inflammatory bowel disease. Alimentary Pharmacology & Therapeutics. 2006;**24**(5):715-729. DOI: 10.1111/j.1365-2036.2006.02980.x

[81] Dubinsky MC, Lamothe S, Yang HY, Targan SR, Sinnett D, Theoret Y, et al. Pharmacogenomics and metabolite measurement for 6-mercaptopurine therapy in inflammatory bowel disease. Gastroenterology. 2000;**118**(4):705-713. DOI: 10.1016/s0016-5085(00)70140-5

[82] Moreau AC, Paul S, Del Tedesco E, Rinaudo-Gaujous M, Boukhadra N, Genin C, et al. Association between 6-thioguanine nucleotides levels and clinical remission in inflammatory disease: A meta-analysis. Inflammatory Bowel Diseases. 2014;**20**(3):464-471. DOI: 10.1097/01.MIB.0000439068.71126.00

[83] Mardini HE, Arnold GL. Utility of measuring 6-methylmercaptopurine and 6-thioguanine nucleotide levels in managing inflammatory bowel disease patients treated with 6-mercaptopurine in a clinical practice setting. Journal of Clinical Gastroenterology. 2003;**36**(5):390-395. DOI: 10.1097/00004836-200305000-00005

[84] Mao R, Guo J, Luber R, Chen BL, He Y, Zeng ZR, et al. 6-Thioguanine nucleotide levels are associated with mucosal healing in patients with Crohn's disease. Inflammatory Bowel Diseases. 2018;**24**(12):2621-2627. DOI: 10.1093/ibd/izy173

[85] Reinshagen M, Schutz E, Armstrong VW, Behrens C, von Tirpitz C, Stallmach A, et al. 6-thioguanine nucleotide-adapted azathioprine therapy does not lead to higher remission rates than standard therapy in chronic active crohn disease: Results from a randomized, controlled, open trial. Clinical Chemistry. 2007;**53**(7):1306-1314. DOI: 10.1373/clinchem.2007.086215

[86] Dassopoulos T, Dubinsky MC, Bentsen JL, Martin CF, Galanko JA, Seidman EG, et al. Randomised clinical trial: Individualised vs. weight-based dosing of azathioprine in Crohn's disease. Alimentary Pharmacology & Therapeutics. 2014;**39**(2):163-175. DOI: 10.1111/apt.12555

[87] Smith M, Blaker P, Patel C, Marinaki A, Arenas M, Escuredo E, et al. The impact of introducing thioguanine nucleotide monitoring into an inflammatory bowel disease clinic. International Journal of Clinical Practice. 2013;**67**(2):161-169. DOI: 10.1111/ijcp.12039

[88] Wright S, Sanders DS, Lobo AJ, Lennard L. Clinical significance of azathioprine active metabolite concentrations in inflammatory bowel disease. Gut. 2004;**53**(8):1123-1128. DOI: 10.1136/gut.2003.032896

[89] Colombel JF, Sandborn WJ, Reinisch W, Mantzaris GJ, Kornbluth A, Rachmilewitz D, et al. Infliximab, azathioprine, or combination therapy for Crohn's disease. The New England Journal of Medicine. 2010;**362**(15):1383-1395. DOI: 10.1056/NEJMoa0904492

[90] Roblin X, Williet N, Boschetti G, Phelip JM, Del Tedesco E, Berger AE, et al. Addition of azathioprine to the switch of anti-TNF in patients with IBD in clinical relapse with undetectable

anti-TNF trough levels and antidrug antibodies: A prospective randomised trial. Gut. 2020;**69**(7):1206-1212. DOI: 10.1136/gutjnl-2019-319758

[91] Ungar B, Kopylov U, Engel T, Yavzori M, Fudim E, Picard O, et al. Addition of an immunomodulator can reverse antibody formation and loss of response in patients treated with adalimumab. Alimentary Pharmacology & Therapeutics. 2017;**45**(2):276-282. DOI: 10.1111/apt.13862

[92] Barnes A, Ooi SJ, Lynch KD, Parthasarathy N, Bishara M, Gounder M, et al. Proactive metabolite testing in patients on Thiopurine may yield long-term clinical benefits in inflammatory bowel disease. Digestive Diseases and Sciences. 2023;**68**(3):889-896. DOI: 10.1007/s10620-022-07556-y

[93] AlAmeel T, Al Sulais E, Raine T. Methotrexate in inflammatory bowel disease: A primer for gastroenterologists. Saudi Journal of Gastroenterology. 2022;**28**(4):250-260. DOI: 10.4103/sjg.sjg_496_21

[94] Feagan BG, Rochon J, Fedorak RN, Irvine EJ, Wild G, Sutherland L, et al. Methotrexate for the treatment of Crohn's disease. The north American Crohn's study group investigators. The New England Journal of Medicine. 1995;**332**(5):292-297. DOI: 10.1056/NEJM199502023320503

[95] Oren R, Arber N, Odes S, Moshkowitz M, Keter D, Pomeranz I, et al. Methotrexate in chronic active ulcerative colitis: A double-blind, randomized, Israeli multicenter trial. Gastroenterology. 1996;**110**(5):1416-1421. DOI: 10.1053/gast.1996.v110.pm8613046

[96] Becher N, Swaminath A, Sultan K. A literature review of Ozanimod therapy in inflammatory bowel disease: From concept to practical application. Therapeutics and Clinical Risk Management. 2022;**18**:913-927. DOI: 10.2147/TCRM.S336139

[97] Colombel JF, Sandborn WJ, Allez M, Dupas JL, Dewit O, D'Haens G, et al. Association between plasma concentrations of certolizumab pegol and endoscopic outcomes of patients with Crohn's disease. Clinical Gastroenterology and Hepatology. 2014;**12**(3):423-31 e1. DOI: 10.1016/j.cgh.2013.10.025

[98] Vande Casteele N, Feagan BG, Vermeire S, Yassine M, Coarse J, Kosutic G, et al. Exposure-response relationship of certolizumab pegol induction and maintenance therapy in patients with Crohn's disease. Alimentary Pharmacology & Therapeutics. 2018;**47**(2):229-237. DOI: 10.1111/apt.14421

[99] Adedokun OJ, Xu Z, Liao S, Strauss R, Reinisch W, Feagan BG, et al. Population pharmacokinetics and exposure-response Modeling of Golimumab in adults with moderately to severely active ulcerative colitis. Clinical Therapeutics. 2020;**42**(1):157-74 e4. DOI: 10.1016/j.clinthera.2019.11.010

[100] Rutgeerts P, Van Assche G, Sandborn WJ, Wolf DC, Geboes K, Colombel JF, et al. Adalimumab induces and maintains mucosal healing in patients with Crohn's disease: Data from the EXTEND trial. Gastroenterology. 2012;**142**(5):1102-11 e2. DOI: 10.1053/j.gastro.2012.01.035

[101] Battat R, Dulai PS, Jairath V, Vande CN. A product review of vedolizumab in inflammatory bowel disease. Human Vaccines & Immunotherapeutics. 2019;**15**(10):2482-2490. DOI: 10.1080/21645515.2019.1591139

[102] Lam MC, Bressler B. Vedolizumab for ulcerative colitis and Crohn's disease: Results and implications of GEMINI studies. Immunotherapy. 2014;**6**(9):963-971. DOI: 10.2217/imt.14.66

[103] Sandborn WJ, Baert F, Danese S, Krznaric Z, Kobayashi T, Yao X, et al. Efficacy and safety of Vedolizumab subcutaneous formulation in a randomized trial of patients with ulcerative colitis. Gastroenterology. 2020;**158**(3):562-72 e12. DOI: 10.1053/j.gastro.2019.08.027

[104] Shmais M, Regueiro M, Hashash JG. Proactive versus reactive therapeutic drug monitoring: Why, when, and how? Inflammatory Intestinal Diseases. 2022;7(1):50-58. DOI: 10.1159/000518755

[105] Sandborn WJ, Feagan BG, Rutgeerts P, Hanauer S, Colombel JF, Sands BE, et al. Vedolizumab as induction and maintenance therapy for Crohn's disease. The New England Journal of Medicine. 2013;**369**(8):711-721. DOI: 10.1056/NEJMoa1215739

[106] Rosario M, French JL, Dirks NL, Sankoh S, Parikh A, Yang H, et al. Exposure-efficacy relationships for Vedolizumab induction therapy in patients with ulcerative colitis or Crohn's disease. Journal of Crohn's & Colitis. 2017;**11**(8):921-929. DOI: 10.1093/ecco-jcc/jjx021

[107] Ward MG, Sparrow MP, Roblin X. Therapeutic drug monitoring of vedolizumab in inflammatory bowel disease: Current data and future directions. Therapeutic Advances in Gastroenterology. 2018;**11**:1756284818772786. DOI: 10.1177/1756284818772786

[108] Williet N, Boschetti G, Fovet M, Di Bernado T, Claudez P, Del Tedesco E, et al. Association between low trough levels of Vedolizumab during induction therapy for inflammatory bowel diseases and need for additional doses within 6 months. Clinical Gastroenterology and Hepatology. 2017;**15**(11):1750-7 e3. DOI: 10.1016/j.cgh.2016.11.023

[109] Benson JM, Peritt D, Scallon BJ, Heavner GA, Shealy DJ, Giles-Komar JM, et al. Discovery and mechanism of ustekinumab: A human monoclonal antibody targeting interleukin-12 and interleukin-23 for treatment of immune-mediated disorders. MAbs. 2011;**3**(6):535-545. DOI: 10.4161/mabs.3.6.17815

[110] Adedokun OJ, Xu Z, Gasink C, Jacobstein D, Szapary P, Johanns J, et al. Pharmacokinetics and exposure response relationships of Ustekinumab in patients with Crohn's disease. Gastroenterology. 2018;**154**(6):1660-1671. DOI: 10.1053/j.gastro.2018.01.043

[111] Battat R, Kopylov U, Bessissow T, Bitton A, Cohen A, Jain A, et al. Association between Ustekinumab trough concentrations and clinical, biomarker, and endoscopic outcomes in patients with Crohn's disease. Clinical Gastroenterology and Hepatology. 2017;**15**(9):1427-34 e2. DOI: 10.1016/j.cgh.2017.03.032

[112] Verstockt B, Dreesen E, Noman M, Outtier A, Van den Berghe N, Aerden I, et al. Ustekinumab exposure-outcome analysis in Crohn's disease only in part explains limited endoscopic remission rates. Journal of Crohn's & Colitis. 2019;**13**(7):864-872. DOI: 10.1093/ecco-jcc/jjz008

[113] Feagan BG, Sandborn WJ, Gasink C, Jacobstein D, Lang Y, Friedman JR, et al. Ustekinumab as induction and maintenance therapy for Crohn's disease. The New England Journal of Medicine. 2016;**375**(20):1946-1960. DOI: 10.1056/NEJMoa1602773

Chapter 6

Predictors of Non-Response to Ongoing Conservative Therapy in Patients with Inflammatory Bowel Disease

Gulustan H. Babayeva, Hikmet I. Ibrahimli, Sergiy V. Holub, Umud R. Mahmudov, Ferid V. Guliyev, Jamal S. Musayev, Emin Kh. Verdiyev, Gunay V. Asadova, Rashad A. Hasanov, Habil M. Huseynov, Aychin I. Hasanova and Tunzala A. Maharramova

Abstract

Crohn's disease (CD) and ulcerative colitis (UC), which are part of the group of inflammatory bowel diseases (IBD), belong to the group of immune-mediated diseases and characterized by a chronic relapsing and chronically continuous course, which leads to serious exacerbations and consequences. Patients may undergo radical surgery, often for drug-resistant disease, and the costs associated with IBD are significant and rising. Over the past two decades, there has been a paradigm shift in the treatment of IBD. The therapeutic goal has shifted from eliminating symptoms alone to achieving combined (symptomatic and endoscopic) remission, which is associated with better outcomes, including a lower risk of relapse, need for corticosteroids, hospitalization, colectomy, and colorectal neoplasia. Despite all the successes, the trend of non-response to ongoing conservative therapy continues. Most studies monitor through endoscopic evaluation and a small number of laboratory tests. There is an important need to understand how noninvasive biomarkers can serve as accurate and reliable indicators for assessing inflammation and predictors of lack of response to therapy. The purpose of this publication is to provide evidence on the use of biomarkers to assess disease activity and predictors of non-response to therapy in patients with IBD.

Keywords: inflammatory bowel disease, ulcerative colitis, Crohn's disease, inflammatory bowel disease, predictors of "non-response", endoscopic activity, pathomorphologic activity, personalized approach

IntechOpen

1. Introduction

Inflammatory bowel diseases are a group of immune-inflammatory pathologies with features of chronicity of the pathological process (chronic recurrent, chronic continuous), with high risks of surgical interventions, malignancy and disability.

Predictors of the lack of a therapeutic response to ongoing conservative therapy may consist of several aspects, first of all, these are the features of the clinical course, endoscopic and histological activity, data from laboratory and imaging diagnostics.

A significant number of individuals with CD need surgical intervention, and 20% of patients with UC undergo proctocolectomy due to resistance to ongoing treatments. The limited research data on indicators for surgery treatment in IBD has led to the initiation of several studies aimed at evaluating risk factors that increase the likelihood of surgery in IBD patients.

In recent years, predictors of non-response to certain drug groups (5-aminosalicylic acid drugs, immunosuppressants, drugs from the genetically engineered therapy group, and so on) have been separately evaluated.

We would like to bring to your attention our mini-review on predictors of non-response to ongoing therapy, markers of aggressive course, as well as a new system for assessing the severity of inflammatory bowel disease, taking into account the marker "influence factor" on the aggravated course and the development of complications.

1.1 What do we know today?

The presence of bleeding, abscesses, fistulas, intestinal obstruction, peritonitis, cases of intestinal perforation and the development of toxic megacolon in this group of patients are urgent circumstances that dictate the need for urgent surgical intervention.

If toxic megacolon is suspected, clinical signs of systemic intoxication in combination with radiological signs (expansion of the diameter of the colon more than 6 cm) are of leading diagnostic importance.

Timely treatment of toxic megacolon begins with intravenous administration of glucocorticoids and antibiotics. However, if there is no significant clinical improvement within the first 3 days in terms of reduction in toxicity and the need for fluid and blood transfusions, resolution of clinical symptoms and normalization of laboratory values, the next step is to consider infliximab or cyclosporine as a drug.

If no improvement is observed after this period of treatment, or if the patient has already received biological therapy, surgical treatment should be immediately considered [1].

Fistulas commonly develop in CD and can be multifaceted, for example between the affected bowel and nearby tissues such as other bowel, bladder, genitals or perianal area. These fistulas can lead to the formation of subcutaneous abscesses. There are various treatment options for fistulas: immunomodulators, biological drugs, antibiotics. However, in cases of lack of therapeutic response to the therapy, the possibility of switching to surgery should be considered [2].

Abscesses usually require antibiotics with percutaneous drainage of abscesses >2 cm in diameter with optimization of Crohn's therapy, but abscess recurrence is possible, so again surgical resection of the affected bowel is often required [2].

Partial or complete intestinal obstruction may be due to the formation of strictures due to severe damage to the lumen of the small intestine with ulceration and transmural inflammation. The stricture becomes symptomatic with superposition of inflammation and spasmodic process. Accordingly, the resulting obstruction can be eliminated by parenteral administration of glucocorticoids, however, in case of acute deterioration, prompt surgical intervention is also required. Fibrous strictures causing recurrent episodes of obstruction should be removed by elective surgery [2].

It is known that the use of biological drugs for treatment can reduce the need for surgery, but despite this, a significant proportion of patients with Crohn's disease, from 60 to 80%, still require surgery. The situation is similar in ulcerative colitis: approximately 20% of patients with ulcerative colitis undergo surgery due to lack of response to previous drug therapy [3].

Some studies have cited high recurrence rates, need for hospitalization, extraintestinal manifestations, multiple hospitalizations for exacerbations, early age at diagnosis, smoking, extensive mucosal ulceration, high serum antibody titers, and NOD2 gene mutations, as predictors of the need for surgery in patients with IBD [4].

In a study by David Marti-Aguado and his colleagues, some important results were obtained [5]:

- The number of patients who did not respond to aminosalicylates was 28%.
- Among patients with a stepped therapy approach, 79% of cases required escalation of treatment within the first 5 years.
- Some predictors of a higher need for therapy have been identified: young age at diagnosis, extensive colitis, endoscopic severity, and the presence of extraintestinal manifestations.
- For those in the step-down group, the reason for escalation was steroid treatment in 76% of cases, steroid resistance in 13%, and extraintestinal manifestations in 5%.
- Increased need for treatment escalation was observed in 97% of patients receiving immunomodulators (IMMs), 57% receiving biological therapy, and 48% of patients receiving a combination of IMM and biological therapy.
- The probability of no need for escalation of therapy after 20 years of follow-up was 65%. Thus, in patients with stepwise treatment, escalation of therapy was observed 2 years after diagnosis, and in 79% of cases, after 5 years of observation, escalation of therapy had already been completed.
- Initial analysis identified several factors that were strongly associated with the need for more intensive treatment: age, dose of 5-ASA, use of a combination approach to treatment, presence of extensive colitis, endoscopic severity of the disease, number of hospitalizations and the occurrence of extraintestinal manifestations (EIM).
- For more potential variables, a multivariate Cox regression model was used to predict the likelihood of switching to escalation therapy: young age, extensive colitis, endoscopic Mayo subscore of 2 or higher, and the presence of extraintestinal manifestations (EIM) were key factors that indicated a higher risk of need escalation of treatment [4] (**Table 1**).

A multivariate logistic regression analysis was conducted to identify factors linked to various escalation strategies, each examined separately and adjusted for

Characteristics	HR (95%CI)	p value
Age at diagnosis	2.31 (1.36–3.92)	<0.01
Disease extent		
• E1, proctitis	Reference	
• E2, left-sided colitis	1.24 (0.75–2.04)	0.40
• E3, extensive colitis	1.65 (1.04–2.60)	0.03
Mayo endoscopic subscore	1.45 (1.02–2.06)	0.04
Baseline 5-ASA dose	0.92 (0.64–1.30)	0.63
Hospitalization	1.68 (0.65–4.31)	0.28
EIMs	2.04 (1.03–4.05)	0.04

5-ASA: 5-aminosalicylate; CI: confidence interval; EIM: extraintestinal manifestations; HR: hazard ratio.

Table 1.
Risk factors for non-response to 5-ASA within 20 years; multivariate cox regression model analysis (HR 95%CI) [4].

gender and disease duration. The utilization of immunomodulatory medications (IMM) and biological agents was found to be associated with several factors, including younger age, extensive colitis, the progression of disease extent, the severity of endoscopic disease, and extraintestinal manifestations (EIMs). Notably, the presence of EIMs at the time of diagnosis was linked to a heightened risk of both IMM (Odds Ratio [OR] 3.69, 95% Confidence Interval [CI] 1.78–7.66) and biological therapy (OR 5.10, 95% CI 2.40–10.85). On the other hand, the development of EIMs during the follow-up period (OR 2.15, 95% CI 1.20–3.86) and the presence of pseudopolyposis (OR 2.13, 95% CI 1.08–4.20) were exclusively associated with the use of IMM. Extensive colitis, prior exposure to IMM, and steroid resistance were significantly correlated with a heightened likelihood of undergoing surgery. The distribution and relationship of disease extension and extent progression with different step-up approaches are detailed in [4] **Table 2**. The authors conducted a subgroup analysis to compare the treatment requirements before and after the introduction of biologic therapies for UC following their approval by the European Medicines Agency in February 2006. The group from the post-biologic

Disease extension	IMM (n = 122)	Biological therapy (n = 72)	Colectomy (n = 16)
E1 (proctitis)	Reference	Reference	n = 0 (0%)
E2 (left-sided)	n = 37 (30%); OR 2.07 (1.04–4.11); p = 0.04	n = 21 (29%); OR 1.77 (0.80–3.70); p = 0.17	Reference
E3 (extensive)	n = 58 (48%); OR 2.93 (1.45–5.89); p < 0.01	n = 33 (46%); OR 2.74 (1.24–6.09); p = 0.02	n = 15 (94%); OR 9.28 (1.14–75.31); p = 0.04
Extent progression	n = 35 (47%); OR 5.19 (2.68–10.04); p < 0.01	n = 23 (31%); OR 4.37 (2.15–8.89); p < 0.01	n = 1 (2%); OR 0.63 (0.07–5.76); p = 0.68

CI: confidence interval; IMM: immunomodulators; OR: odds ratio.

Table 2.
Multivariate logistic regression analysis showing association of disease extension and extent progression with different step-up approaches (expressed as: n (%); OR (95% CI); p value). Bold values indicate they are statistically significant [4].

era (comprising 246 individuals) showed a notable decrease in the rates of colectomy (7% vs. 1%; $p < 0.01$) when compared to the pre-biologic era. Among the individuals who followed a step-up treatment approach, only 21% required treatment escalation within a 5-year follow-up period. Within this cohort, the authors conducted a subgroup analysis, which demonstrated the absence of any kind of significant divergences between patients who required treatment escalation within a relatively short period (≤5 years, n = 99) and those who had a longer time before requiring treatment escalation (>5 years, n = 27).

Previously published studies have identified several risk factors for relapse and the need for colectomy. These include younger age, male gender, shorter disease duration, smoking, extensive colitis, and initial low hemoglobin levels (<10.5 g/dL) in patients primarily treated with 5-ASA medication [6–10]. When examining factors associated with the use of a step-up treatment approach, the authors' data support the findings related to younger age and extensive colitis, consistent with previous research. However, in contrast to the relapse rate, the researchers did not observe any differences based on gender or smoking habits. It's worth noting that a recent meta-analysis also found that smokers did not experience significantly fewer disease flares [11]. The association between age and non-response to 5-ASA aligns with other studies that have shown younger patients are more likely to require steroids or experience a shorter time to relapse [6, 12], ultimately leading to a lower age at which treatment escalation becomes necessary. Similarly, the relationship between the Mayo endoscopic subscore and the adoption of a step-up approach suggests that the severity of the initial disease might serve as a significant predictor of unfavorable treatment outcomes.

A study by Carsten Schmidt et al. showed that, this study identifies anemia and an early need for corticosteroids as predictors for a complicated course of disease in an inception cohort of patients with UC. By determining these parameters in routine clinical practice, our results may support the identification of patients who might benefit from early escalation of therapy [13] and a Risk Model was built to predict the complicated course of the disease (**Table 3**).

In a study by Elena De Cristofaro and colleagues [14], other predictors for surgery were identified: low serum albumin levels and colonic dilatation in patients with acute severe ulcerative colitis (ASUC) who respond to intravenous corticosteroid therapy (IV CS) or treatment with infliximab (IFX). ASUC is characterized by severe flare-ups in approximately one-fourth of individuals with ulcerative colitis (UC), as defined by the Truelove and Witts criteria [15–17]. For those who do not respond to IV CS within 3-5 days, second-line treatments like cyclosporine or infliximab (IFX) are considered rescue options [18]. Although these interventions have significantly improved the outlook for patients with IV CS-refractory UC, particularly in terms of reducing the need for colectomy, more than one-fourth of patients still require urgent colectomy [19]. Multiple predictors of colectomy have been identified in this subset of ASUC patients. These factors encompass clinical characteristics (such as gender, stool frequency, prior exposure to biological therapies, and steroid dependence), biological indicators (including albumin, C-reactive protein [CRP], and hemoglobin levels), as well as endoscopic and radiographic findings (such as the presence of "mucosal islands" and colonic dilation) [19–22]. Additionally, superinfections like *Clostridium difficile* and *Cytomegalovirus* have been recognized as additional prognostic factors [23, 24].

In patients with acute severe ulcerative colitis (ASUC) who show a positive response to intravenous corticosteroids (IV CS) or infliximab (IFX) during their initial hospitalization, the likelihood of requiring colectomy tends to rise if they experience a second hospitalization for ASUC [25]. Specifically, individuals who do not fully

Time	Corticosteroids	Anemia	Probability of IS, %
After 6 months	No	No	10.5
	Yes	No	15.1
	No	Yes	13.7
	Yes	Yes	19.6
After 12 months	No	No	17.0
	Yes	No	24.0
	No	Yes	21.9
	Yes	Yes	30.7
After 24 months	No	No	23.0
	Yes	No	32.1
	No	Yes	29.5
	Yes	Yes	40.3

Table 3.
Risk model for prediction of complicated disease course [13].

respond to steroid treatment have a 50% chance of needing colectomy within 1 year after being discharged, and this risk escalates to 70% within 5 years [26].

To address this concern, a recent scoring system was developed with the aim of distinguishing ASUC patients at low risk from those at high risk of undergoing colectomy within 1 year following hospitalization. This scoring system took into account previous exposure to TNF antagonists or thiopurines, the presence of *Clostridium difficile* infection, and serum levels of C-reactive protein (CRP) and albumin as predictive factors for colectomy. However, it's worth noting that the aforementioned ranking system lacked radiological and endoscopic criteria, and the follow-up period after hospitalization was relatively short [27]. Consequently, the common knowledge of the factors predicting long-term colectomy in ASUC patients who have achieved a complete clinical response to medical therapy remains limited.

A rather interesting and timely review on predictors of non-response in ulcerative colitis was presented in 2015 by a group of researchers led by Cláudia Camila Dias [28]. Potential predictors of colectomy included such indicators as gender, degree of disease, smoking history, hospitalization and the need for treatment with corticosteroids at any stage of the course of ulcerative colitis (UC). Utilizing a random effects model, our analysis revealed that female patients exhibited a reduced risk of colectomy (Odds Ratio [OR] 0.78, 95% Confidence Interval [CI] 0.68 to 0.90). Importantly, there was no significant evidence of statistical heterogeneity (I2 = 49%) in aforementioned findings, as illustrated in [28] (**Figure 1**). The random effects model showed that patients with extensive disease had a higher risk of colectomy (OR 3.68 [95% CI 2.39, 5.69]); however, significant heterogeneity was found among them (I^2 = 67%) [28] (**Figure 2**).

Regarding smoking habits, the analysis using a random effects model indicated that individuals who smoked had a reduced risk of requiring colectomy (OR 0.55 [95% CI 0.33 to 0.91]). Importantly, there was no notable heterogeneity in these findings (I^2 = 0%) [28] (**Figure 3**).

Patients who experienced hospitalization at any point in their disease course faced an elevated risk of undergoing colectomy, as indicated by the analysis

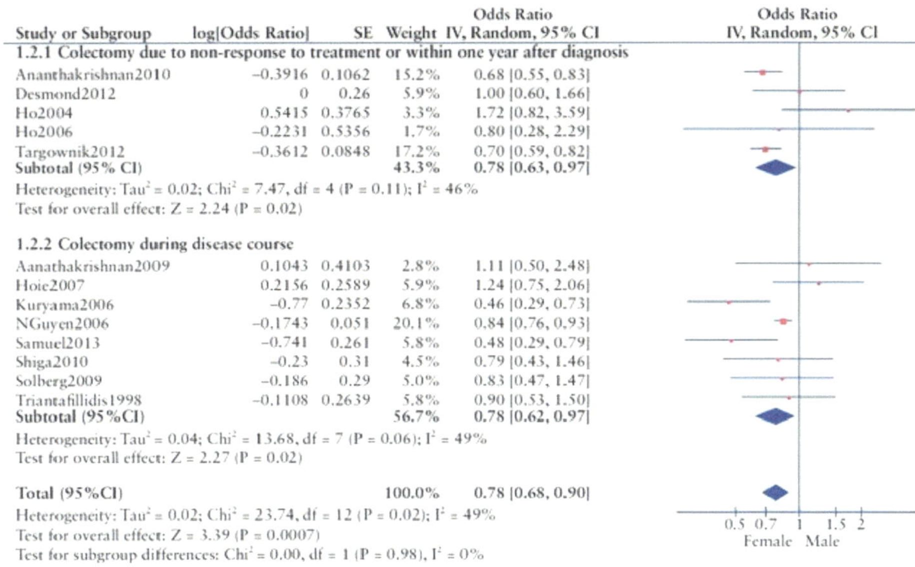

Figure 1.
Gender as a predictor of colectomy [28].

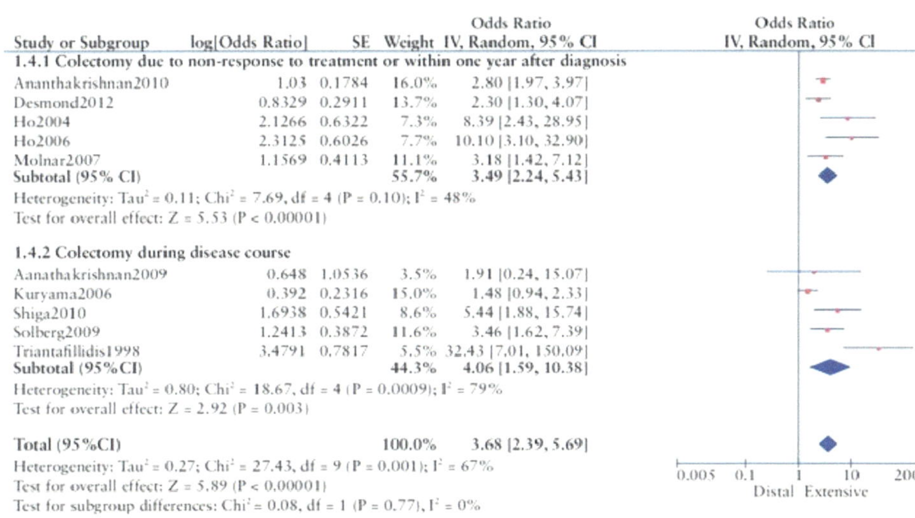

Figure 2.
Disease extent as a predictor of colectomy [28].

(OR 4.13 [95% CI 3.23, 5.27]). Notably, the authors' findings did not reveal any significant evidence of statistical heterogeneity (I^2 = 0%) [28] (**Figure 4**).

An association between the use of corticosteroids and colectomy was found in four studies. Patients who took corticosteroids (oral or intravenous) at any time had a higher risk of colectomy (OR 2.10 [95% CI 1.05, 4.22]); however, significant heterogeneity was found (I^2 = 54%) [28] (**Figure 5**).

The authors [28] performed a subgroup analysis focusing on two colectomy outcomes: due to lack of response to treatment/or within the first year after diagnosis and colectomy occurring throughout the disease. In this analysis, the factors influencing

Study or Subgroup	log[Odds Ratio]	SE	Weight	Odds Ratio IV, Random, 95% CI
1.5.1 Colectomy due to non-response to treatment or within one year after diagnosis				
Ho2004	−0.7557	0.8322	9.7%	0.47 [0.09, 2.40]
Ho2006	−0.821	1.1096	5.5%	0.44 [0.05, 3.87]
Subtotal (95% CI)			**15.2%**	**0.46 [0.12, 1.69]**
Heterogeneity: Tau² = 0.00; Chi² = 0.00, df = 1 (P = 0.96); I² = 0%				
Test for overall effect: Z = 1.17 (P = 0.24)				
1.5.2 Colectomy during disease course				
Aanathakrishnan2009	−0.8873	0.6329	16.8%	0.41 [0.12, 1.42]
Hoie2007	−0.4273	0.3905	44.2%	0.65 [0.30, 1.40]
Solberg2009	−0.6162	0.5329	23.7%	0.54 [0.19, 1.53]
Subtotal (95%CI)			**84.8%**	**0.56 [0.32, 0.98]**
Heterogeneity: Tau² = 0.00; Chi² = 0.39, df = 2 (P = 0.82); I² = 0%				
Test for overall effect: Z = 2.03 (P = 0.04)				
Total (95%CI)			**100.0%**	**0.55 [0.33, 0.91]**
Heterogeneity: Tau² = 0.00; Chi² = 0.48, df = 4 (P = 0.98); I² = 0%				
Test for overall effect: Z = 2.32 (P = 0.02)				
Test for subgroup differences: Chi² = 0.08, df = 1 (P = 0.77), I² = 0%				

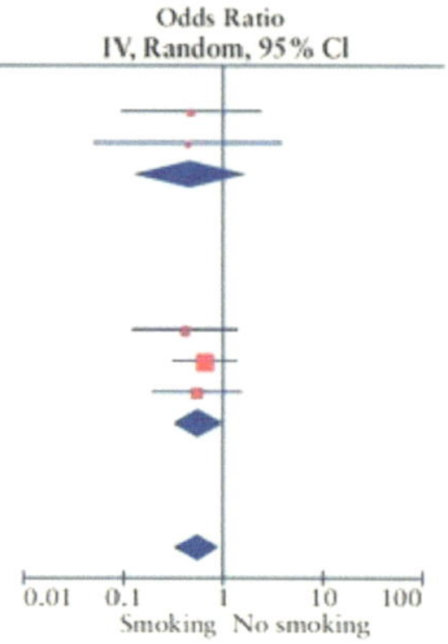

Figure 3.
Smoking habits as a predictor of colectomy [28].

Study or Subgroup	log[Odds Ratio]	SE	Weight	Odds Ratio IV, Random, 95% CI
Aanathakrishnan2009	1.766	1.0536	1.4%	5.85 [0.74, 46.11]
Desmond2012	1.2809	0.2911	18.3%	3.60 [2.03, 6.37]
Targownik2012	1.4436	0.1391	80.3%	4.24 [3.23, 5.56]
Total (95%CI)			**100.0%**	**4.13 [3.23, 5.27]**
Heterogeneity: Tau² = 0.00; Chi² = 0.36, df = 2 (P = 0.83); I² = 0%				
Test for overall effect: Z = 11.38 (P < 0.00001)				

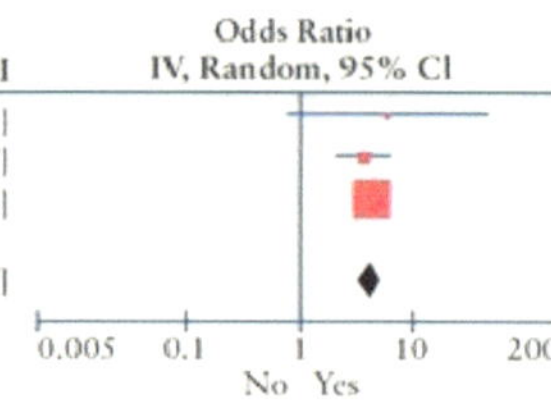

Figure 4.
Hospitalization as a predictor of colectomy [28].

Study or Subgroup	log[Odds Ratio]	SE	Weight	Odds Ratio IV, Random, 95% CI
Desmond2012	0.2624	0.3158	35.1%	1.30 [0.70, 2.41]
Ferrante2008	0.8754	0.398	30.2%	2.40 [1.10, 5.24]
Hefti2009	2.182	0.7424	15.6%	8.86 [2.07, 37.98]
Ho2004	0.2479	0.6322	19.1%	1.28 [0.37, 4.42]
Total (95%CI)			**100.0%**	**4.13 [3.23, 5.27]**
Heterogeneity: Tau² = 0.26; Chi² = 6.47, df = 3 (P = 0.09); I² = 54%				
Test for overall effect: Z = 2.09 (P = 0.04)				

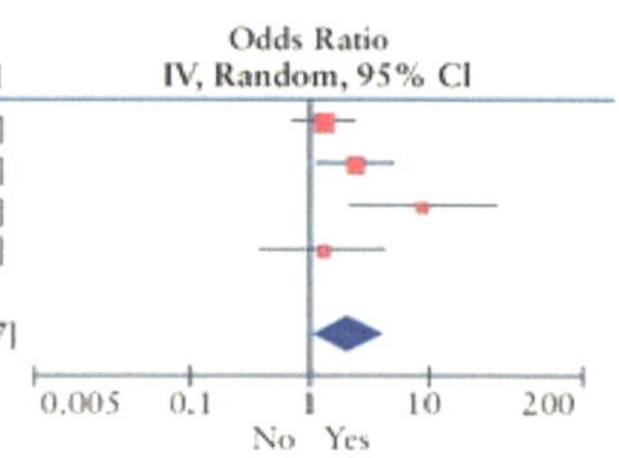

Figure 5.
Use of the corticosteroids as a predictor of colectomy [28].

these results were: gender, degree of disease, smoking. Returning to earlier data that controlled for gender (**Figure 1**), extent of disease (**Figure 2**), and smoking habit (**Figure 3**), no significant differences in the likelihood of undergoing surgery, regardless of its nature, occurring within the first year after surgery were found diagnosis or at a later stage of the disease.

In evaluating C-reactive protein (CRP) as a potential prognostic factor for colectomy, the authors [28] encountered challenges from the seven studies reviewed that presented different risk estimates, differences in timing of CRP measurement, and different cutoff values for risk assessment. These discrepancies prevented data from being combined for analysis.

None of three separate investigations [29–34] has provided the median or mean CRP levels. Furthermore, none of these studies disclosed the specific method used for measuring CRP levels, which posed a challenge in arriving at any meaningful conclusions. With the exception of one study [29], all the others exhibited a noticeable trend where individuals with elevated CRP levels were more likely to undergo colectomy. Ho GT et al. [32] introduced a risk index to assist in identifying patients who did not respond to treatment, leading to colectomy. They observed that non-responders had higher CRP levels compared to responders (6.9 mg/L versus 3.9 mg/L, p 4 weeks after the first induction therapy (HR 1.15 [95% 0.82, 1.62]). In a study by patients requiring colectomy [33], those admitted with elevated CRP values had significantly higher levels than their counterparts (mean [standard deviation] of 116 [102] versus 43 [25] mg/L). Similarly, Lindgren et al. [34] identified CRP levels of ≥25 mg/L on the third day of hospitalization as a predictor of colectomy within the first 30 days of hospital stay. Colectomized patients also exhibited notably higher CRP levels on the third day after treatment compared to non-colectomized patients (36.3 mg/L versus 18.0 mg/L, with a p-value of 0.007). Furthermore, one-year post-diagnosis, patients with CRP levels ≥10 mg/L faced a significantly elevated risk of undergoing colectomy in the subsequent 4 years, with an odds ratio of 3.0 [95% confidence interval: 1.1, 7.8] [35]. Regarding the timing of infliximab induction, two studies reported an association between elevated CRP values and an increased risk of colectomy. One study observed this association at CRP levels ≥10 mg/L, with a hazard ratio of 5.11 [95% confidence interval: 1.77, 14.76] [31], while the other study noted it at CRP levels ≥5 mg/L, with a hazard ratio of 14.5 [95% confidence interval, 2.0, 108.6] [30].

There are several compelling reasons why prognostic factors hold significant importance in the context of UC management, for instance [36]:

1. Mucosal healing has become a crucial therapeutic goal in UC management [16, 37];

2. The introduction of drugs from the group of biological therapies, such as anti-tumor necrosis factor medications, which has opened up possibilities for promoting mucosal healing and sustaining prolonged clinical remission in UC patients [38]; and

3. The lead of early therapeutic interventions to more favorable outcomes in UC patients [16, 37].

Given these imperatives, it becomes paramount to develop a specialized clinical tool capable of assessing disabilities and identifying specific factors that can predict UC outcomes. Therefore, the clinical risk factors analyzed in aforementioned meta-analysis should be taken into account when creating new scoring systems or approaches for evaluating UC outcomes. The authors highlight certain characteristics that can aid healthcare professionals in identifying risk groups among UC patients. This represents a significant stride in establishing predictive factors for UC, demonstrating their practicality and influence on disease prognosis, particularly the risk of colectomy. Factors such as gender, disease extent, hospitalization history, the need for corticosteroid treatment, smoking habits, and CRP levels were found to be associated with the likelihood of colectomy. Although there are other markers that can assist clinicians in forecasting the course of UC, including genetic, serologic, and endoscopic findings, the authors' meta-analysis has specifically focused on demographic and clinical characteristics. This choice was made due to the ease of assessing these factors at the time of diagnosis and during routine patient care. As for CRP, variations in risk estimation methods and inadequate information regarding measurement techniques precluded authors from combining the data for analysis.

Nonetheless, a notable trend emerged suggesting an increased risk of colectomy among patients with elevated CRP (C-reactive protein) levels. Among the findings, the most significant risk factors identified in this analysis were the presence of extensive disease, hospitalization and smoking habits. According to the research outcomes from subgroups within the patient population, the predictors for colectomy remained consistent whether it was due to nonresponse to treatment at the time of diagnosis or within the first year after diagnosis, or occurred during the course of the disease. Gender, disease extent, and smoking habits continued to show strong associations, emphasizing their importance in predictive models. The researchers attempted to assess factors like multiple hospitalizations per year and recurrent flares requiring steroid treatment as indicators of chronic morbidity. However, there was insufficient data in the studies for a comprehensive analysis of these factors. Additionally, the authors could not explore the roles of other clinical and demographic variables, such as age at diagnosis, either because the data were unavailable or because they could not be aggregated due to variations in measurement methods. Furthermore, the authors encountered limitations in the analysis of several clinical trials involving UC due to the absence of stratified outcomes, specifically regarding gender, disease extent, smoking habits, hospitalization rates, and the necessity for corticosteroids. The majority of the studies included in authors' analysis were of good quality; however, they did identify shortcomings in how outcomes were adjusted for in four of them. The primary limitation researches encountered in their meta-analysis was the presence of heterogeneity among the studies, stemming from differences in their methodologies and approaches. To gauge the impact of this heterogeneity on authors' results, they conducted a sensitivity analysis. The aforementioned analysis indicated that their findings remained relatively stable, suggesting that the results are robust and dependable. Nevertheless, it's important to acknowledge these limitations when interpreting the results and drawing conclusions.

In summary, the mentioned-above review and meta-analysis have underscored the significance of certain clinical factors, including gender, disease extent, smoking habits, hospitalization, and the use of corticosteroids, in predicting the outcome of ulcerative colitis, particularly the risk of colectomy. Integrating these parameters into the development of predictive models for UC prognosis holds the potential to improve the clinical approach and enhance the outcomes for patients dealing with severe forms of the disease.

Another rather interesting study was carried out by Egyptian colleagues [39], which studied predictors of surgery in patients with inflammatory bowel disease.

This study encompassed 80 individuals diagnosed with IBD, falling within an age range of 34 to 65 years. Among them, 40 were male, and 29 were smokers. The average age at which the disease first manifested was approximately 25.81 ± 6.8 years, with half of the patients experiencing involvement solely in the colon, while about 33.75% had both colonic and small intestinal complications. Extraintestinal symptoms, such as uveitis, arthritis, and arthralgia, were present in 61.3% of cases, and 37.5% of patients had perianal issues, with 27.5% showing granulomas in their histopathological reports. The mean Clinical Disease Activity Index (CDAI) score for Crohn's disease (CD) patients was 298.45 ± 83.3, and for those with ulcerative colitis (UC), the mean Mayo score was 8.65 ± 1.9 [39].

Within the group of 40 patients who underwent surgical procedures, 30% had UC, while 70% had CD. Among these surgical cases, the procedures included total colectomy (30%), fistulectomy (32.5%), resection anastomosis (17.5%), and abdominal abscess drainage (20%). Patients in the surgical group exhibited a higher prevalence of perianal disease and smoking. Additionally, the CDAI scores for CD patients and the Mayo scores for UC patients were notably higher in the surgical group (P value <0.001). Crohn's disease and the presence of granulomas were more frequently observed in the surgical group (P value <0.05). Conversely, factors such as the age of disease onset, the location of the disease, and the presence of extraintestinal manifestations did not show any statistically significant differences when comparing both patient groups (P value >0.5) [39].

In the group of patients who underwent surgery, there were notable differences in certain medical markers compared to the non-surgical group. Specifically, surgical patients exhibited significantly higher levels of stool calprotectin (P value <0.001), CRP (P value <0.001), and erythrocyte sedimentation rate (ESR) (P value <0.001). Additionally, CD patients in the surgical group had lower serum albumin levels at the onset of the disease compared to their non-surgical counterparts (P value <0.001). However, there were no significant differences observed in terms of complete blood count (CBC) parameters between the two groups, as indicated in [39] (**Table 4**).

Cutoff values, sensitivity, and specificity of significant scores and laboratory parameters are attached in [39] **Table 5**.

There are numerous viable treatments available for IBD, such as Crohn's disease and ulcerative colitis. However, a portion of individuals either do not respond well to

Variable	Group 1 Mean ± SD	Group 2 Mean ± SD	*P* value
Stool Calprotectin level (μg/g)	543.35 ± 210.1	342.12 ± 229.2	<0.001
CRP level (mg/dl)	67.57 ± 14.1	33.35 ± 10.6	<0.001
Albumin level at time of diagnosis (g/dl) for CD	3.10 ± 0.42	4.62 ± 0.39	<0.001
ESR(mm/h)	59.95 ± 5.1	30.75 ± 4.1	<0.001
Hemoglobin (g/dL)	10.14 ± 0.59	9.87 ± 0.63	0.058
Hematocrit %	35.9 ± 2.9	36.32 ± 2.9	0.52
White blood cells (×1000 cell/mm^3)	12.25 ± 0.9	14.3 ± 1.4	0.41
Platelet count (×1000 cell/mm^3)	519.2 ± 54.3	498.42 ± 44.3	0.064

SD standard deviation.

Table 4.
Comparison between both groups as regard laboratory data [39].

Variables	Surgical TTT			
	Cutoffs	Sensitivity	Specificity	Value
CDAI for CD	>287	90%	85%	0.01
Mayo score for UC	>8.5	90%	70%	0.01
Stool calprotectin level (μg/g)	>341.5	92.5%	78.5%	0.01
CRP (mg/dl)	>44	99%	87.5%	0.01
ESR (mm/h)	>55	92.5%	100%	0.01

Table 5.
Cutoff values of different scores and inflammatory markers in prediction of surgical intervention in IBD patients [39].

these treatments initially or eventually lose their positive response [40]. In such cases, when the disease becomes medically refractory, surgical procedures like intestinal resection or proctocolectomy may become necessary [16].

It is crucial to identify patients who are at a high likelihood of needing surgery for Inflammatory Bowel Disease (IBD). However, the ability to predict which patients will require surgical intervention is still not well-established. To address this issue, a comparative study involving two medical centers was conducted in Egypt, involving 80 patients with IBD. The primary goal was to identify the factors that increase the risk of surgical intervention in these IBD patients.

It is crucial to identify patients who are at a high likelihood of needing surgery for IBD. However, the ability to predict which patients will require surgical intervention is still not well-established. To address this issue, a comparative study involving two medical centers was conducted in Egypt, involving 80 patients with IBD. The primary goal was to identify the factors that increase the risk of surgical intervention in these IBD patients.

Regarding the age of disease onset, the study found that the average age was 25.81 years, with a standard deviation of 6.8 years. This finding aligns with a study by De Barros et al. [41], which also analyzed the epidemiological characteristics of 40 IBD patients undergoing biologic therapy. In their retrospective observational clinical study, they observed a similar trend where the average age of disease onset was around 25 years old.

In the presented study, the authors showed that, the most prevalent site of the disease in IBD patients was the colon. This finding is consistent with the study conducted by Lehtinen et al. [42], which also pointed to the colon as the most frequently affected location. Moreover, Aziz et al. [43] conducted a 5-year retrospective study to assess various clinical presentations of IBD and similarly found that the colon was the most commonly affected site.

This study's results showed that there was no statistically significant difference in the age at which the disease began between patients who required surgery and those who underwent medical treatment (P value = 0.37). This aligns with the findings of Lee et al. [12], who reported that the rates of surgery were not significantly linked to the age of onset in Korean ulcerative colitis patients. Additionally, a larger North American registry study also demonstrated that the age at which UC begins does not correlate with the likelihood of surgical intervention [44].

In this investigation, authors observed that smoking was significantly more prevalent among patients in group 1 ($P < 0.001$), and this was identified as a predictor of surgical treatment. This observation is in line with the research conducted by Karczewski et al. [45], who explored the impact of tobacco use on the clinical course of IBD.

In this study, authors [39] observed that extraintestinal manifestations were present in 61.3% of the cases, which closely resembles the findings of the study by de Barros et al. [41], where extraintestinal manifestations were noted in 70% of the patients. However, in this research, despite being more prevalent in Crohn's disease (CD) patients, there was no statistically significant difference between those who required surgery and those treated medically in terms of extraintestinal manifestations ($P = 0.25$). This contrasts with a retrospective analysis of endoscopic balloon dilatation of intestinal strictures in CD, which reported that the presence of extraintestinal manifestations and extensive preoperative disease were more likely to necessitate further dilatation or surgery following an initial dilatation [46]. It's possible that these differences can be attributed to variations in the ethnic backgrounds of the study populations.

Authors identified statistically significant differences between patients who underwent surgery and those who received medical treatment based on the type of IBD. Specifically, CD patients were more prevalent than UC patients in group 1 ($P = 0.02$). Surgical patients were also more likely to have perianal disease ($P < 0.01$) and granulomas ($P < 0.012$). These findings are consistent with research conducted by Nasir et al. [47], who documented that perianal disease and the presence of the NOD2 genotype were the only independent factors associated with the need for surgery. Similarly, Agar et al. [48] revealed that the presence of complicated disease features at the time of diagnosis, such as intestinal stenosis and fistulas, were independent predictive risk factors for subsequent surgery in CD patients.

Authors [39] observed statistically significant differences in disease activity scores between the two groups. Specifically, for Crohn's disease patients, the Crohn's Disease Activity Index (CDAI) was significantly higher (P value <0.001), and for ulcerative colitis patients, the Mayo score was also significantly higher (P value <0.001) in group 1, which included patients requiring surgery. Notably, CDAI scores greater than 287 and Mayo scores exceeding 8.5 demonstrated high sensitivity and specificity in identifying patients who needed surgical treatment. These findings align with research conducted by Agar et al. [48], who reported that a CDAI score above 250 was an independent predictive risk factor for future surgery in CD patients.

Furthermore, this study found that the mean levels of C-reactive protein (CRP) were 50.46 ± 21.2 (mg/dl), indicating elevated CRP levels. Similarly, the mean erythrocyte sedimentation rate (ESR) and white blood cell (WBC) count were 45.35 ± 15.4 mm/h and $13.28 \pm 10.9 \times 1000$ cell/mm^3, respectively, indicating increased expression of these biomarkers. These observations are in agreement with the findings of Alper et al. [49], who conducted research correlating ESR and CRP levels with the diagnosis of IBD and with disease activity assessed through clinical, endoscopic, histological, and radiographic measures. They found that IBD patients consistently exhibited significantly higher ESR and leukocyte counts. Solem et al. [50] also supported these findings in their research, highlighting the elevated levels of these biomarkers in IBD patients.

Analysis in this study [39] revealed statistically significant differences between patients who underwent surgery and those treated medically regarding C-reactive protein (CRP) levels (P value <0.001) and erythrocyte sedimentation rate (ESR) (P value <0.001). In group 1, which included patients requiring surgery, both CRP and ESR levels were notably higher. Specifically, a CRP level above 44 mg/dL was identified as a predictor of the need for surgical treatment, with a high sensitivity of 99% and specificity of 87.5%. These findings are consistent with a prospective study conducted in Oxford that assessed severe ulcerative colitis patients, where CRP levels exceeding 45 mg/L were a strong indicator (85% certainty) of the requirement for colectomy [33]. Additionally, Henriksen et al. [51] investigated the predictive value of CRP levels in UC patients with extensive colitis and found that CRP levels above 23 mg/L at diagnosis were associated with an increased risk of surgery. Similarly, in patients with Crohn's disease, a significant association was found between CRP levels at diagnosis and the risk of surgery, with CRP levels above 53 mg/L indicating an elevated risk [51].

Authors [39] also assessed stool calprotectin levels as a predictor of surgical treatment. A stool calprotectin level greater than 341.5 μg/g was identified as a predictor, with a high sensitivity of 92.5% and specificity of 78.5%. These findings align with the work of Kennedy et al. [52], who reported that an increased level of fecal calprotectin during the initial visit was associated with the subsequent progression of CD and the need for surgery. Calprotectin concentration in UC patients was also found to correlate with worse outcomes, including the need for surgery [53]. Theede et al. [54] demonstrated that in UC, a baseline stool calprotectin level exceeding 321 μg/g predicted unfavorable outcomes, including the requirement for surgery.

In conclusion, the Egyptian researchers found that several factors were linked to an increased risk of requiring surgical intervention in patients with IBD. These factors encompassed smoking habits, the presence of Crohn's disease, perianal complications, the development of granulomas, elevated severity scores (such as CDAI and Mayo score), higher levels of stool calprotectin, increased C-reactive protein levels, and elevated erythrocyte sedimentation rates. Furthermore, they identified smoking, perianal disease, CDAI, Mayo score, stool calprotectin level, C-reactive protein level, and erythrocyte sedimentation rate as valuable predictors of the need for surgical treatment, as these factors exhibited strong statistical significance in patients who ultimately required surgical intervention [39].

Considering the variations observed in assessing predictors of non-response in patients with Inflammatory Bowel Disease (IBD), including the disease's aggressiveness, we have reached the conclusion that the essential laboratory diagnostics used in the daily practice of specialists dealing with IBD should be reevaluated. While C-reactive protein and calprotectin are currently considered mandatory markers, we believe that it's worth exploring additional laboratory parameters.

With this in mind, our study aimed to develop a monitoring system for evaluating the condition of IBD patients, taking into account a broader range of laboratory tests.

2. Materials and methods

In the period from August 2015 to June 2022, 388 patients with a diagnosis of IBD. The diagnosis of IBD was made following widely accepted criteria, in line with the guidelines provided by the European Crohn's and Colitis Organization (ECCO) [55, 56]. To evaluate the disease's clinical severity, we used established measures such as the Truelove-Witts Index (TW) and Mayo score for ulcerative colitis, and the Crohn's Disease Activity Index (CDAI) and Harvey-Bradshaw index (HBI) for Crohn's disease.

The study [57, 58] did not include patients with severe cardiac and nephrological pathology, as well as those who underwent surgery within the last 6 months or are in the stage of clinical and endoscopic remission. Thus, the study included 250 patients; of these, 112 (44.8%) had CD and 138 (55.2%) UC. The age of patients was from 18 to 60 years (39.4 ± 4.6), by gender: 129 (51.6%) women and 121 (48.4%) men. The duration of the disease before contacting a specialist doctor was 1.1-8.3 years (3.7 ± 1.2), patients were under dynamic observation from 6 to 48 months (18.4 ± 7.2). In addition to the general clinical examination, the following laboratory markers were obligatory determined: highly sensitive C-reactive protein (h/s-CRP), homocysteine, vitamin D, platelet level, eosinophilic catthione protein, α-TNF, IL-1β, IL-2, IL-4, IL-6, IL-8, IL-10, IL-18 in blood, calprotectin, lactoferrin and TM-2-pyruvate kinase (TM2-P) in feces, albumin level (micro- and macro) in urine. Patients, if necessary, underwent repeated studies (680 cases in total). In our statistical analysis of the collected data, we employed standard descriptive statistical methods, including calculating the arithmetic mean (M), standard deviation (σ), and standard error (m) for the measured characteristics. When comparing numerical values between different groups, we utilized Student's t-coefficient, and we determined the probability of error (p). To explore the relationships between various indicators, we calculated the Pearson correlation coefficient (®).

3. Results of the study and their discussion

The results obtained during the study are presented in [57, 58] **Table 6**.

We conducted separate analyses for the detection of each of these indicators in both the ulcerative colitis (UC) and Crohn's disease (CD) groups, but no significant differences were observed ($p > 0.05$). Similarly, when we examined the results based on gender, there were no significant differences ($p > 0.05$).

Number of studies laboratory indicator	CD (n = 325)	UC (n = 355)	Total (n = 680)
High Sensitivity CRP: (N 1-3 mg/L)	*325 (100%)*	*355 (100%)*	*680 (100%)*
before 3 mg/L	11 (3.4%)	17 (4.8%)	28 (4.1%)
from 3 to 10 mg/L	106 (32.6%)	98 (27.6%)	204 (30%)
from 10 to 20 mg/L	74 (22.7%)	127 (35.8%)	201 (29.5%)
from 20 to 30 mg/L	95(29.2%)	87(24.5%)	182 (26.7%)
more 30 mg/L	39 (12%)	26 (7.3%)	65 (9.6%)
Homocysteine: (N < 12 μmol/L)	*325 (66.7%)*	*355 (69%)*	*680 (67.9%)*
before 12 μmol/L	108 (33.3%)	110 (30.9%)	218 (32%)
from 12 to 16 μmol/L f	83 (25.5%)	97 (27.3%)	180 (26.5%)
from 16 to 20 μmol/L	52 (16%)	63 (17.7%)	115 (16.9%)
from 20 to 24 μmol/L	48 (14.7%)	49 (13.8%)	97 (14.3%)
more 24 μmol/L	34 (10.5%)	36 (10.1%)	70 (10.3%)
Vitamin D: (N > 30 ng/mL)	*325 (100%)*	*355 (100%)*	*680 (100%)*
30–20 ng/mL	108 (33.2%)	121 (34.1%)	75 (21.1%)
20–10 ng/mL	159 (48.9%)	174 (49%)	172 (48.6%)
less 10 ng/mL	58 (17.8%)	60 (16.9%)	106 (30.0%)
Platelets: (N 150,000–400,000/mm³)	*325 (76%)*	*355 (74.3%)*	*680 (72.0%)*
before 400,000/mm³	78 (24%)	91 (25.6%)	169 (24.8%)
from 400,000 to 440,000/mm³	101 (31%)	124 (34.9%)	225 (33%)
from 440,000 to 480,000/mm³	92 (28.3%)	101 (28.4%)	193 (28.4%)
from 480,000 to 520,000/mm³	33 (10.2%)	28 (7.9%)	61 (9%)
more 520,000/mm³	21 (6.5%)	11 (3.1%)	32 (4.7%)
Fecal calprotectin (N < 50 μg/g)	*325 (96.6%)*	*355 (93.8%)*	*680 (95.1%)*
before <50 μg/g	11 (3.4%)	22 (6.2%)	33 (4.8%)
from 50 to 150 μg/g	43 (13.2%)	29 (8.2%)	72 (10.6%)
from 150 to 250 μg/g	77 (23.7%)	59 (16.6%)	136 (20%)
from 250 to 500 μg/g	83 (25.5%)	95 (26.7%)	178 (26.2%)
more 500 μg/g	111 (34.1%)	150 (42.3%)	261 (38.4%)
Fecal lactoferrin (N < 7.25 μg/g)	*325 (97.8%)*	*355 (98.3%)*	*680 (98%)*
before <7.25 μg/g	7 (2.2%)	6 (1.7%)	13 (19.1%)
from 7.25 to 14.5 μg/g	46 (14.2%)	55 (15.5%)	101 (14.8%)
from 14.5 to 22 μg/g	87 (26.7%)	91 (25.6%)	178 (26.2%)

Number of studies laboratory indicator	CD (n = 325)	UC (n = 355)	Total (n = 680)
from 22 to 29.5 μg/g	90 (27.7%)	100 (28.2%)	190 (27.9%)
more 29.5 μg/g	95(29.2%)	103 (29%)	198 (29.1%)
Fecal TM-2-pyruvate kinase (N < 4 U/ml)	*325 (98.2%)*	*355 (98.9%)*	*680 (98.5%)*
before <4 U/ml	6 (1.8%)	4 (1.1%)	10 (1.5%)
from 4 to 6 U/ml	28 (8.61%)	34 (9.6%)	62 (9.1%)
from 6 to 10 U/ml	65 (20%)	72 (20.3%)	137 (20.1%)
from 10 to 20 U/ml	83 (25.5%)	99 (27.9%)	182 (27.8%)
more 20 U/ml	143 (44%)	146 (41.1%)	289 (42.5%)
a-TNF (N 4.6–12.4 pg/ml)	*325 (97.2%)*	*355 (98.6%)*	*680 (97.9%)*
from 0 to 4.6 pg/ml	9 (2.7%)	5 (1.4%)	14 (2%)
from 4.6 to 12.4 pg/ml	13 (4%)	19 (5.4%)	32 (4.7%)
from 12.4 to 25 pg/ml	70 (21.5%)	84 (23.6%)	154 (22.6%)
from 25 to 35 pg/ml	94 (28.9%)	102 (28.7%)	196 (28.8%)
более 35 pg/ml	139 (42.7%)	145 (40.8%)	284 (41.8%)
IL-1β (N < 11 pq/ntl)	24 (7.4%)	33 (9.3%)	57 (8.4%)
IL-2 (N < 10 pq/ml)	19 (5.8%)	26 (7.3%)	45 (6.6%)
IL-4 (N < 4 pq/ml)	13 (4%)	17 (4.8%)	30 (4.4%)
IL-6 (N < 10 pq/ml)	37 (11.4%)	41 (11.6%)	78 (11.5%)
IL-8 (N < 10 pq/ml)	119 (36.6%)	137 (38.6%)	256 (37.6%)
IL-10 (N < 20 pq/ml)	82 (25.2%)	88 (24.8%)	170 (25%)
IL-18 (N < 261 pq/ml)	69 (21.2%)	73 (20.6%)	142 (20.9%)
Albumin in urine	152 (46.7%)	175 (49.3%)	327 (48%)
Microalbuminuria (less 30 mg/L)	108 (33.2%)	124 (38.2%)	232 (34.1%)
Macroalbuminuria (more than 30 mg/L)	44 (13.5%)	51 (14.4%)	95 (13.9%)

Table 6.
Distribution of studied parameters in patients with ulcerative colitis and Crohn's disease [57, 58].

To explore a potential relationship between endothelial dysfunction indicators and the patients' conditions, as per recommended guidelines, we conducted computer-based data processing. The severity of changes in these studied endothelial dysfunction indicators was evaluated as a percentage relative to the permissible range of the normal values. This assessment considered both increases in the indicator beyond the upper limit of the norm and decreases below the lower limit. The results of this analysis are presented in [57, 58] **Table** 7.

Our findings indicate that the severity of endothelial dysfunction, categorized between 4 to 6 points, corresponds to a mild clinical course of Inflammatory Bowel Disease (IBD). A score ranging from 6 to 9 points suggests a moderate level of severity, and if the score exceeds 9 points, it indicates a high degree of clinical disease severity. Clinical and endoscopic remission, on the other hand, corresponds to a score of 3 points or less. The degree of correlation between these indicators was found to be 0.863.

Currently, the diagnosis of IBD relies on protocols that encompass a comprehensive assessment, including clinical evaluation, instrumental procedures, laboratory

Laboratory indicator/ Severity	Norm	I degree (mild)	II degree (medium-severe)	III degree (severe)
h/s CRP	N	1.3 N	1.5 N	>1.5 N
Homocysteine	N	1.3 N	1.5 N	>1.5 N
Platelets	N	1.1 N	1.2 N	>1.2 N
Vitamin D	N	0.7 N	0.4 N	<0.4 N
Fecal calprotectin	N	2 N	3 N	>3 N
Albumin in urine	N	—	Micro-	Macro-
Points	0	1	2	3

Table 7.
Correlation of some indicators of endothelial dysfunction, inflammation and the severity of the clinical course in patients with inflammatory bowel disease [57, 58].

tests, and pathological examinations. Instrumental studies primarily emphasize radiation-based imaging methods such as CT, MRI, and ultrasound, along with thorough endoscopic examinations involving multiple biopsies from at least five sections of the intestine. In laboratory diagnostics, in addition to routine assessments and the exclusion of opportunistic infections, the determination of fecal calprotectin (a marker of intestinal mucosal damage) in stool samples has gained importance. Recently, the assessment has extended to include fecal lactoferrin and the acute-phase inflammation marker, C-reactive protein (CRP), in blood tests.

While the current diagnostic approach offers clear advantages, it comes with two notable drawbacks: high costs associated with the study and delays in diagnosis due to the need for pathomorphological examination results. Another critical factor is patient compliance with diagnostic procedures like MRI, CT scans, and endoscopy. In contrast, laboratory diagnostics primarily rely on just two indicators: calprotectin levels in stool samples and CRP levels in blood tests.

The literature extensively discusses the potential for incorporating additional laboratory diagnostic methods [59–62]. When choosing a range of laboratory tests, we proceeded from the fact that IBD is based on immunological, aseptic inflammation. It is known that any inflammation is a manifestation of dysfunction of endothelial cells, which are involved in all phases of acute and chronic inflammation [60]. Endothelial cells play a crucial role in creating a barrier between the bloodstream and body tissues. They also produce various factors that serve vital regulatory functions, contributing to the maintenance of overall bodily balance (homeostasis). It is widely acknowledged that endothelial dysfunction (ED) is a typical pathological process and a central factor in the development of numerous diseases and their associated complications, including IBD. In the context of IBD, the inflammatory process within the intestinal mucosa, particularly the infiltration of leukocytes, can damage the endothelial cells lining the blood vessels in the intestinal mucosa. This damage can lead to disturbances in microcirculation, the formation of microthrombi, and subsequent trophic changes. Currently, several parameters are examined to assess endothelial dysfunction. These include homocysteine levels, thrombocytosis, von Willebrand factor, endothelin, highly sensitive C-reactive protein (CRP), changes in lipid profiles, interleukin patterns, plasminogen activator inhibitor-1 (PAI-1), plasminogen activator inhibitor-2 (PAI-2), intercellular adhesion molecule-1 (ICAM-1), nitric oxide (NO), P- and E-selectins, among others. Additionally, recent research has identified vitamin D deficiency as a risk factor for the development of autoimmune conditions [60].

We have selected the most accessible, both in practical (availability/availability in the laboratory network) and in economic terms, studies of indicators of endothelial dysfunction and immuno-allergic changes. These indicators were: homocysteine, platelets, highly sensitive CRP, eosinophilic cationic protein and vitamin D in the blood, fecal calprotectin, lactoferrin and tumor 2-pyruvate kinase, as well as microalbumin in the urine [57, 58].

Our findings lead us to the conclusion that the severity of certain markers of endothelial dysfunction, as well as immune-allergic changes, directly correlates with the severity of a patient's condition. However, it's important to note that since there is no significant difference observed between the patient groups with ulcerative colitis (UC) and Crohn's disease (CD), these changes exhibit a low level of specificity. Consequently, they are best applied in cases where a diagnosis has already been established.

The advantages of utilizing this approach include:

1. **Economic feasibility:** It is a cost-effective method.

2. **Speed of calculation:** Results can be obtained quickly.

3. **Ease of implementation for the patient:** The procedure is relatively simple for patients to undergo.

4. **Widespread availability in outpatient practice:** This method is readily accessible for use in outpatient healthcare settings.

4. Conclusion

Thus, in addition to the already existing predictors of lack of response to ongoing therapy, taking into account clinical, endoscopic, laboratory activity, we can add the extended laboratory diagnostics of IBD that we proposed, which allows, with an established diagnosis, not to resort to repeated expensive studies and obtain results in real time, allowing personalize the assessment of the severity of the patient's condition. This allows you to create an individual system for monitoring the patient's condition, make timely decisions on the need for additional studies and correction of therapy, which is especially important in outpatient practice in matters of identifying a lack of response to ongoing conservative treatment.

Conflict of interest

The author affirms that there are no conflicts of interest to disclose.

Author details

Gulustan H. Babayeva[1*], Hikmet I. Ibrahimli[2], Sergiy V. Holub[3], Umud R. Mahmudov[4], Ferid V. Guliyev[5], Jamal S. Musayev[6], Emin Kh. Verdiyev[7], Gunay V. Asadova[1,5], Rashad A. Hasanov[1,8], Habil M. Huseynov[9], Aychin I. Hasanova[1] and Tunzala A. Maharramova[1,5]

1 Department of Therapy, Azerbaijan State Advanced Training Institute for Doctors named after A. Aliyev, Baku, Azerbaijan

2 Department of Health Organization, Azerbaijan State Advanced Training Institute for Doctors named after A. Aliyev, Baku, Azerbaijan

3 Department of Software of Automated Systems, Cherkasy State Technological University, Cherkassy, Ukraine

4 Department of Gastroenterology and Endoscopy, Modern Hospital, Baku, Azerbaijan

5 Department of Invasive Diagnosis and Treatment, National Centre of Oncology, Baku, Azerbaijan

6 Department of Pathomorphology, Baku Pathology Center, Baku, Azerbaijan

7 Department of Gastroenterology and Endoscopy, Central Hospital, Baku, Azerbaijan

8 Department of Gastroenterology and Endoscopy, German Hospital, Baku, Azerbaijan

9 Department of Gastroenterology and Endoscopy, Oncology Clinic, Azerbaijan Medical University, Baku, Azerbaijan

*Address all correspondence to: ghbabayeva@gmail.com

References

[1] Sheth SG, LaMont JT. Toxic megacolon. Diseases of the Colon and Rectum. 2019;**51**(8):1283-1291

[2] Pfefferkorn MD, Marshalleck FE, Saeed SA, Splawski JB, Linden BC, Weston BF. NASPGHAN clinical report on the evaluation and treatment of pediatric patients with internal penetrating Crohn disease: Intraabdominal abscess with and without fistula. Journal of Pediatric Gastroenterology and Nutrition. 2013;**57**(3):394-400. DOI: 10.1097/MPG.0b013e31829ef850

[3] Lightner AL. Surgery for inflammatory bowel disease in the era of biologics. Journal of Gastrointestinal Surgery. 2020;**24**:1430-1435

[4] Yarur AJ, Strobel SG, Deshpande AR, Abreu MT. Predictors of aggressive inflammatory bowel disease. Gastroenterología y Hepatología. 2011;**7**:652-659

[5] Marti-Aguado D, Ballester MP, Tosca J, Bosca-Watts MM, Navarro P, Anton R, et al. Long-term follow-up of patients treated with aminosalicylates for ulcerative colitis: Predictive factors of response: An observational case-control study. United European Gastroenterology Journal. 2019;**7**(8):1042-1050. DOI: 10.1177/2050640619854277

[6] Bitton A, Peppercorn MA, Antonioli DA, et al. Clinical, biological, and histologic parameters as predictors of relapse in ulcerative colitis. Gastroenterology. 2001;**120**:13-20

[7] Lee HJ, Jung ES, Lee JH, et al. Long-term clinical outcomes and factors predictive of relapse after 5-aminosalicylate or sulfasalazine therapy in patients with mild-to-moderate ulcerative colitis. Hepato-Gastroenterology. 2012;**59**:1415-1420

[8] Bello C, Belaiche J, Louis E, et al. Evolution and predictive factors of relapse in ulcerative colitis patients treated with mesalazine after a first course of corticosteroids. Journal of Crohn's & Colitis. 2011;**5**:196-202

[9] Garcia-Planella E, Mañosa M, Van Domselaar M, et al. Long-term outcome of ulcerative colitis in patients who achieve clinical remission with a first course of corticosteroids. Digestive and Liver Disease. 2012;**44**:206-210

[10] Höie O, Wolters F, Riis L, et al. Ulcerative colitis: Patient characteristics may predict 10-yr disease recurrence in a European-wide population-based cohort. The American Journal of Gastroenterology. 2007;**102**:1692-1701

[11] To N, Ford AC, Gracie DJ. Systematic review with meta-analysis: The effect of tobacco smoking on the natural history of ulcerative colitis. Alimentary Pharmacology & Therapeutics. 2016;**44**:117-126

[12] Lee J, Cheon J, Moon C, et al. Do patients with ulcerative colitis diagnosed at a young age have more severe disease activity than patients diagnosed when older? Digestion. 2010;**81**:237-243

[13] Schmidt C, Bokemeyer B, Lügering A, Bettenworth D, Teich N, Fischer I, et al. Clinical predictors for a complicated course of disease in an inception cohort of patients with ulcerative colitis: Results from the prospective, observational EPICOL study. International Journal of Colorectal Disease. 2022;**37**:485-493

[14] De Cristofaro E, Salvatori S, Marafini I, Zorzi F, Alfieri N, Musumeci M, et al. Long-term risk of colectomy in patients with severe ulcerative colitis responding to intravenous corticosteroids or infliximab. Journal of Clinical Medicine. 2022;**11**(6):1679. DOI: 10.3390/jcm11061679]

[15] Truelove SC, Witts LJ. Cortisone in ulcerative colitis: Final report on a therapeutic trial. British Medical Journal. 1955;**2**:1041-1048

[16] Turner D, Walsh CM, Steinhart AH, Griffiths AM. Response to corticosteroids in severe ulcerative colitis: A systematic review of the literature and a meta-regression. Clinical Gastroenterology and Hepatology. 2007;**5**:103-110

[17] Turner D, Walsh CM, Benchimol E, Mann EH, Thomas KE, Chow C, et al. Severe paediatric ulcerative colitis: Incidence, outcomes and optimal timing for second-line therapy. Gut. 2008;**57**:331-338

[18] Narula N, Marshall J, Colombel J-F, Leontiadis GI, Williams JG, Muqtadir Z, et al. Systematic review and meta-analysis: Infliximab or cyclosporine as rescue therapy in patients with severe ulcerative colitis refractory to steroids. The American Journal of Gastroenterology. 2016;**111**:477-491

[19] Järnerot G, Hertervig E, Friis-Liby I, Blomquist L, Karlén P, Grännö C, et al. Infliximab as rescue therapy in severe to moderately severe ulcerative colitis: A randomized, placebo-controlled study. Gastroenterology. 2005;**128**:1805-1811

[20] Ventham NT, Kalla R, Kennedy NA, Satsangi J, Arnott ID. Predicting outcomes in acute severe ulcerative colitis. Expert Review of Gastroenterology & Hepatology. 2015;**9**:405-415

[21] Lynch RW, Churchhouse AMD, Protheroe A, Arnott IDR. The UK IBD audit steering group. Predicting outcome in acute severe ulcerative colitis: Comparison of the Travis and Ho scores using UK IBD audit data. Alimentary Pharmacology & Therapeutics. 2016;**43**:1132-1141

[22] Shah SC, Colombel J-F, Sands BE, Narula N. Mucosal healing is associated with improved long-term outcomes of patients with ulcerative colitis: A systematic review and meta-analysis. Clinical Gastroenterology and Hepatology. 2016;**14**:1245-1255

[23] Law CCY, Tariq R, Khanna S, Murthy S, McCurdy JD. Systematic review with meta-analysis: The impact of Clostridium difficile infection on the short- and long-term risks of colectomy in inflammatory bowel disease. Alimentary Pharmacology & Therapeutics. 2017;**45**:1011-1020

[24] Ananthakrishnan AN, McGinley EL, Binion DG. Excess hospitalisation burden associated with Clostridium difficile in patients with inflammatory bowel disease. Gut. 2008;**57**:205-210

[25] Dinesen LC, Walsh AJ, Protic MN, Heap G, Cummings F, Warren BF, et al. The pattern and outcome of acute severe colitis. Journal of Crohn's and Colitis. 2010;**4**:431-437

[26] Bojic D, Radojicic Z, Nedeljkovic-Protic M, Al-Ali M, Jewell DP, Travis SP. Long-term outcome after admission for acute severe ulcerative colitis in Oxford: The 1992-1993 cohort. Inflammatory Bowel Diseases. 2009;**15**:823-828

[27] Le Baut G, Kirchgesner J, Amiot A, Lefevre JH, Chafai N, Landman C, et al. A scoring system to determine patients' risk of colectomy within 1 year after hospital admission for

acute severe ulcerative colitis. Clinical Gastroenterology and Hepatology. 2021;**19**:1602-1610.e1

[28] Dias C, C, Rodrigues PP, da Costa-Pereira A, Magro F. Clinical predictors of colectomy in patients with ulcerative colitis: Systematic review and meta-analysis of cohort studies. Journal of Crohn's and Colitis. Feb 2015;**9**(2):156-163. DOI: 10.1093/ecco-jcc/jju016

[29] Shiga H, Takagi S, Inoue R, et al. What determines the later clinical course of patients who do not undergo colectomy at the first attack? A Japanese cohort study on ulcerative colitis. Digestion. 2010;**81**:104-112

[30] Ferrante M, Vermeire S, Fidder H, et al. Long-term outcome after infliximab for refractory ulcerative colitis. Journal of Crohn's & Colitis. 2008;**2**:219-225

[31] Oussalah A, Evesque L, Laharie D, et al. A multicenter experience with infliximab for ulcerative colitis: Outcomes and predictors of response, optimization, colectomy, and hospitalization. The American Journal of Gastroenterology. 2010;**105**:2617-2625

[32] Ho GT, Mowat C, Goddard CJR, et al. Predicting the outcome of severe ulcerative colitis: Development of a novel risk score to aid early selection of patients for second-line medical therapy or surgery. Alimentary Pharmacology & Therapeutics. 2004;**19**:1079-1087

[33] Travis SPL, Farrant JM, Ricketts C, et al. Predicting outcome in severe ulcerative colitis. Gut. 1996;**38**:905-910

[34] Lindgren SC, Flood LM, Kilander AF, Löfberg R, Persson TB, Sjödahl RI. Early predictors of glucocorticosteroid treatment failure in severe and moderately severe attacks of ulcerative colitis. European Journal of Gastroenterology & Hepatology. 1998;**10**:831-835

[35] Henriksen M, Jahnsen J, Lygren I, et al. C-reactive protein: A predictive factor and marker of inflammation in inflammatory bowel disease. Results from a prospective population-based study. Gut. 2008;**57**:1518-1523

[36] Devlin SM, Panaccione R. Evolving inflammatory bowel disease treatment paradigms: Top-down versus step-up. The Medical Clinics of North America. 2010;**94**:1-18

[37] Magro F, Rodrigues-Pinto E, Coelho R, et al. Is it possible to change phenotype progression in Crohn's disease in the era of immunomodulators? Predictive factors of phenotype progression. The American Journal of Gastroenterology. 2014;**109**:1026-1036

[38] Latella G, Papi C. Crucial steps in the natural history of inflammatory bowel disease. World Journal of Gastroenterology. 2012;**18**:3790-3799

[39] El Megeed KHA, Saleh SAB, Mohamed AE, Anwar CA. Predictors of surgical intervention in patients with inflammatory bowel disease (two-center study). The Egyptian Journal of Internal Medicine. 2021;**33**:19

[40] Hazel K, O'Connor A. Emerging treatments for inflammatory bowel disease. Therapeutic Advances in Chronic Disease. 2020;**11**:204062231989929. DOI: 10.1177/2040622319899297

[41] de Barros PAC, da Silva AMR, Lins Neto MÂDF. Perfilepidemiológico dos pacientesportadores de doença inflamatória intestinal, Que fazemuso da terapiabiológica, Atendidosem um hospital da rede pública de alagoas. Journal of Coloproctology. 2014;**34**:131-135

[42] Lehtinen P, Ashorn M, Iltanen S, Jauhola R, Jauhonen P, Kolho KL, et al. Incidence trends of pediatric inflammatory bowel disease in Finland, 1987-2003, a nationwide study. Inflammatory Bowel Diseases. 2011;**17**(8):1778-1783. DOI: 10.1002/ibd.21550]

[43] Aziz DA, Moin M, Majeed A, Sadiq K, Biloo AG. Paediatric inflammatory bowel disease: Clinical presentation and disease location. Pak Journal of Medical Sciences. 2017;**33**:793-797

[44] Hyams J, Markowitz J, Lerer T, Griffiths A, Mack D, Bousvaros A, et al. The natural history of corticosteroid therapy for ulcerative colitis in children. Clinical Gastroenterology and Hepatology. 2006;**4**(9):1118-1123. DOI: 10.1016/j.cgh.2006.04.008]

[45] Karczewski J, Poniedzialek B, Rzymski P, Rychlewska Hańczewska A, Adamski Z, Wiktorowicz K. The effect of cigarette smoking on the clinical course of inflammatory bowel disease. Archive of "Przeglad Gastroenterologiczny". 2014;**9**:153-159

[46] Gustavsson A, Magnuson A, Blomberg B, Andersson M, Halfvarson J, Tysk C. Smoking is a risk factor for recurrence of intestinal stricture after endoscopic dilation in Crohn's disease. Alimentary Pharmacology & Therapeutics. 2013;**37**(4):430-437. DOI: 10.1111/apt.12176]

[47] Nasir BF, Griffiths L, Nasir A, Roberts R, Barclay M, Gearry R, et al. Perianal disease combined with NOD2 genotype predicts need for IBD-related surgery in Crohn's disease patients from a population-based cohort. Journal of Clinical Gastroenterology. 2013;**47**(3):242-245. DOI: 10.1097/MCG.0b013e318258314d]

[48] Agar K, Medhioub M, Jardak S, Hamzaoui L, Khsiba A, Azzouz MM. P418 predictive factors of surgery in the course of Crohn's disease. Journal of Crohn's & Colitis. 2018;**12**(supplement_1):S315-S316. DOI: 10.1093/ecco-jcc/jjx180.545

[49] Alper A, Zhang L, Pashankar DS. Correlation of erythrocyte sedimentation rate and C-reactive protein with pediatric inflammatory bowel disease activity. Journal of Pediatric Gastroenterology and Nutrition. 2017;**65**(2):e25-e27. DOI: 10.1097/MPG.0000000000001444

[50] Solem CA, Loftus EV, Tremaine WJ, Harmsen WS, Zinsmeister AR, Sandborn WJ. Correlation of C-reactive protein with clinical, endoscopic, histologic, and radiographic activity in inflammatory bowel disease. Inflammatory Bowel Diseases. 2005;**11**:707-712

[51] Henriksen M, Jahnsen J, Lygren I, Stray N, Sauar J, Vatn MH, et al. C-reactive protein: A predictive factor and marker of inflammation in inflammatory bowel disease. Results from a prospective population-based study. Gut. 2008;**57**:1518-1523

[52] Kennedy NA, Jones GR, Plevris N, Patenden R, Arnott ID, Lees CW. Association between level of fecal calprotectin and progression of Crohn's disease. Clinical Gastroenterology and Hepatology. 2019;**17**:2269-76.e4. DOI: 10.1016/j.cgh.2019.02. 017

[53] Guirgis M, Wendt E, Wang LM, Walsh A, Burger D, Bryant RV, et al. Beyond histological remission: Intramucosal calprotectin as a potential predictor of outcomes in ulcerative colitis. Journal of Crohn's & Colitis. 2017;**11**:460-467

[54] Theede K, Holck S, Ibsen P, Kallemose T, Nordgaard-Lassen I, Nielsen AM. Fecal calprotectin predicts relapse and histological mucosal healing in ulcerative colitis. Inflammatory Bowel Diseases. 2016;**22**(5):1042-1048. DOI: 10.1097/MIB.0000000000000736

[55] Harbord M, Eliakim R, et al. 3rd European evidence-based consensus on diagnosis and management of ulcerative colitis. Part 2. Journal of Crohn's and Colitis. 1 Jul 2017;**11**(7):769-784. DOI: 10.1093/ecco-jcc/jjx009

[56] Gomollón F, Dignass A, et al. 3rd European evidence-based consensus on the diagnosis and management of crohn's disease 2016: Part 1. Journal of Crohn's and Colitis. Jan 2017;**11**(1):3-25. DOI: 10.1093/ecco-jcc/jjw168

[57] Babayeva GH, Babayev ZM. New approach to the estimation of a clinical flow in patients with ulcerative colitis and Crohn's disease. Experimental and Clinical Gastroenterology. 2019;**162**(2):19-23. (In Russ.). DOI:10.31146/1682-8658-ecg-162-2-19-23

[58] Babayeva GH, Babayev ZM. Frequency of detection of some markers of endothelial dysfunction in patients with inflammatory bowel diseases. Terapevticheskiy arxiv. 2018;**4**:12-16 (In Russ.). DOI: 10.26442/terarkh201890412-16

[59] Derkacz A, Olczyk P, Komosinska-Vassev K. Diagnostic markers for nonspecific inflammatory bowel diseases. Disease Markers. 2018;(5):1-16. DOI: 10.1155/2018/7451946

[60] Babayeva GH, Samedova TA, Babayev ZM, Huseynova FR. On the role of vitamin D deficiency in some pathological conditions. Saglamliq. 2018;(2):23-32 (In Russ.)

[61] Barnes EL et al. New biomarkers for diagnosing inflammatory bowel disease and assessing treatment outcomes. Inflammatory Bowel Diseases. 2016;**22**(12):2956-2965. DOI: 10.1097/MIB.0000000000000903

[62] Norouzinia M, Chaleshi V, et al. Biomarkers in inflammatory bowel diseases: Insight into diagnosis, prognosis and treatment. Gastroenterology and Hepatology from Bed to Bench. 2017;**10**(3):155-167

Chapter 7

Surgical Interventions in Inflammatory Bowel Disease

Bahadir Kartal

Abstract

Inflamatuar bowel disease represent a disease spectrum with protean manifestation and complications. Although as many as half of the patients with inflammatory bowel disease require at least one surgical procedure during their lifetime, the decision to operate is rarely an easy one. Such a decision should be the result of collaboration between the gastroenterologist and the surgeon, assisted by the radiologist and the pathologist. The age and general conditions of the patient, the extent of disease, the duration of disease and prior treatment, as well as any specific complication must be considered in making the decision. Surgical interventions in Crohn's disease are usually performed in patients who develop complications or have symptoms that are resistant to drug therapy. Surgical treatment is not curative, it is aimed at minimizing the disease. Ulcerative colitis surgery, on the other hand, is examined as an emergency and elective. Once the need for surgical intervention has been established, other factors, specific to the individual, must be considered to choose the most appropriate surgical procedure.

Keywords: Crohn's disease, ulcerative colitis, surgery, indeterminate colitis, inflamatuar bowel disease

1. Introduction

Inflammatory bowel diseases (IBD) represent a complex disease spectrum, showcasing a multitude of clinical manifestations and potential complications. Deciding to proceed with surgical intervention in IBD cases is a nuanced process, demanding a collaborative effort involving gastroenterologists, surgeons, radiologists, and pathologists. Several critical factors, such as the patient's age, overall health, extent and duration of the disease, prior treatment history, and the presence of specific complications, must be meticulously considered in the decision-making process. Upon confirming the necessity for surgical intervention, it becomes imperative to customize the surgical procedure based on the individual patient's unique characteristics and needs.

2. Crohn's disease

Crohn's disease is a chronic, diffuse condition that has the potential to affect all segments of the gastrointestinal system, characterized by recurrent flare-ups and for which surgical cure is not attainable. Surgical intervention becomes imperative

IntechOpen

when conservative medical therapy proves ineffective or when patients develop complications such as spontaneous bowel perforation, intestinal obstruction, profuse hemorrhage, and severe inflammatory responses, such as acute fulminant colitis, necessitating immediate surgical management [1]. Additionally, patients with Crohn's disease may encounter chronic complications like recurrent bowel obstructions and neoplastic growths, both of which can serve as indications for surgical intervention (**Table 1**). Nevertheless, it is worth noting that the determination of appropriate surgical indications and the optimal timing for surgical intervention remain subjects of ongoing debate.

2.1 Fistula

The association between fistulas and Crohn's disease is unsurprising, given the transmural inflammatory nature of the condition. Fistulas can manifest either in the early postoperative phase, within weeks following surgery, or at a later stage. Fistulas can present as either internal or external, with internal fistulas potentially arising as enteroenteric connections or extending from the bowel to various adjacent structures or organs, including but not limited to the bladder, vagina, or retroperitoneum. Enterocutaneous fistulas are categorized as external fistulas. Frequently, a stenotic region in the bowel wall is found distal to the point of fistula origin, leading to an elevation in intraluminal pressure. This particular scenario increases the predisposition to the development of such fistulas [2]. Low-output fistulas, especially in patients at high surgical risk, should be approached with non-surgical methods. If surgery is deemed necessary, resection should involve the portion of the diseased or obstructed segment proximal to the fistula. Performing wedge resection or strictureplasty within the fistula-containing segment is not recommended, as it may lead to postoperative leakage and fistula recurrence [3]. In cases of complicated fistula in a patient with widespread enterolysis, multiple anastomoses, closure of enterotomies, and procedures such as strictureplasty, the creation of a diverting ileostomy from a proximal location is warranted. Enteroenteric fistulas represent the prevailing form of abdominal fistulas encountered in Crohn's disease, with the majority originating from the terminal ileum. These fistulas initiate within the affected segment of the bowel; nevertheless, they possess the capacity to penetrate into adjacent normal tissue. Ileosigmoid fistula is the most prevalent among this category of fistulas. Standard treatment approaches for these cases involve the removal of the diseased bowel,

Fistula
Abscesses
Obstruction
Hemorrhage
Cancer
Failure of medical therapy
Perforation
Toxic colitis

Table 1.
Indications for surgery in Crohn's disease.

excision or division of the fistula tract, and the repair of the non-inflamed bowel wall. Additionally, some patients may manifest with a psoas abscess, resulting from a blind-ending fistula originating from the ileum and extending into the retroperitoneum. The management of such cases necessitates the excision of the inflamed bowel to address the condition and forestall its recurrence [4]. Enteroenteric fistulas represent the prevailing type of abdominal fistula observed in the context of Crohn's disease, predominantly originating from the terminal ileum. These fistulas have their onset within the affected bowel segment; however, they possess the capacity to breach the boundaries into adjacent normal tissue. The standard approach for managing these cases typically involves the resection of the diseased bowel, excision or separation of the fistula tract, and restoration of the non-inflamed bowel wall. Additionally, some patients may present with a psoas abscess, which results from a blind-ending fistula extending from the ileum into the retroperitoneal space. In such instances, the resolution and prevention of recurrence necessitate the excision of the inflamed bowel [5]. Enterocutaneous fistulas can manifest either spontaneously or as a consequence of prior surgical procedures. These fistulas can significantly impact patients by causing dehydration, metabolic disturbances, skin damage, and disruptions in daily life due to uncontrolled discharge. The etiology of these fistulas plays a critical role in determining the most appropriate treatment and the likelihood of success. Approximately 75–85 percent of enterocutaneous fistulas occur in the postoperative period and are often linked to anastomotic leaks or inadvertent bowel injuries. Given the healthy nature of the affected bowel in these cases, conservative measures are more likely to lead to fistula closure. On the other hand, 15–25 percent of enterocutaneous fistulas are spontaneous and typically arise from diseased bowels affected by conditions like Crohn's disease, radiation damage, or cancer. Surgical intervention is usually necessary for the closure of such fistulas [6, 7]. In fistula surgery, following the resection of the diseased segment and subsequent anastomosis, the primary repair of the fistula opening in adjacent organs (e.g., stomach, duodenum, bladder, vagina, and sigmoid colon) is recommended. Resection of the adjacent organ related to the fistula is only warranted if that organ is affected by Crohn's disease. Bridging should be avoided, as it can perpetuate the disease in the bridged area, leading to potential complications such as abscess formation, bleeding, perforation, and bacterial contamination [8].

2.2 Abscesses

The formation of an abscess arises due to a microperforation stemming from the transmural inflammation of the affected bowel. The predominant anatomical site within the abdominal cavity where these abscesses tend to develop is the ileocecal region [5]. Psoas abscess emerges due to retroperitoneal perforation in the ileocecal region. Clinical presentations range from mild sepsis to pronounced psoas spasm, characterized by hip pain, thigh flexion, and external thigh rotation, often accompanied by the presence of an abdominal mass. Typically, relief is achieved through the resection of the inflammatory mass and drainage of the abscess. When practicable, it is advisable to handle these patients through a regimen involving image-guided drainage and antibiotics, reserving elective resection for a subsequent juncture. This strategy proves viable for approximately half of the patient population [9]. Technical success is achieved in more than 90% of percutaneous drainage procedures, and in the short term, over 50% of patients can circumvent the necessity for surgery [10]. In cases involving multiple abscesses, the likelihood of necessitating surgical intervention is higher. Surgical intervention becomes imperative if the patient either does not respond to drainage or fails to show improvement. In cases where the extent of the inflammatory response is extensive and encompasses multiple adjacent bowel loops, the approach should be primarily focused on abscess drainage and the establishment of a proximal diverting stoma. The primary objective of the procedure should be the drainage of the abscess, resolution of sepsis, and resection of the affected intestinal segment. Subsequently, if the patient's hemodynamic and nutritional status permit and the final suture line can be placed at a distance from the abscess cavity, a primary anastomosis can be constructed. It is also prudent to apply an omental flap onto the remaining wall of the abscess cavity to isolate any lingering infection from the abdominal cavity and the anastomosis. If a primary anastomosis is not deemed advisable, the creation of a temporary end ileostomy becomes necessary. Subsequently, after the acute inflammatory reaction has largely subsided, a selective resection of the affected bowel can be undertaken, thus preserving a substantial portion of the bowel that might otherwise have been resected during the initial exploration. Abdominal wall abscesses, including iliopsoas and rectus sheath abscesses, are relatively less common, with an estimated prevalence falling within the range of 0.4–4%. Nevertheless, it is noteworthy that they present a more formidable challenge in terms of control when compared to intra-abdominal abscesses [9].

2.3 Obstruction

Around 20–25% of Crohn's disease surgeries are necessitated by obstruction-related issues [11]. Patients often present with episodic crampy abdominal pain and abdominal distention. Subsequent recurrent acute episodes can exacerbate the scarring process, resulting in the formation of a fibrotic stricture and a potential escalation in symptom severity. Additional causes of obstruction in Crohn's disease patients encompass anastomotic strictures and cancers. Chronic small bowel obstructions can arise from either singular or multiple strictures, which may be either short or long in length. Patients afflicted by this condition typically exhibit symptoms such as postprandial abdominal pain, nausea, and vomiting, which can gradually escalate into a high-grade obstruction. In cases where multiple constrictive strictures exist, the small bowel undergoes a transformation, assuming the form of a series of dilated saccular segments interspersed by constrictive, ring-like strictures. The expanded segments, characterized by the presence of partially digested food particles, create a conducive environment for bacterial overgrowth. Due to this bacterial overgrowth and the resultant stasis, patients frequently report symptoms such as intermittent diarrhea, malabsorption issues. If there are multiple strictures in the intestine, they can only be resolved through resection [12]. In selected cases, balloon dilation and stricturoplasty are preferred methods for managing intestinal strictures. The choice of strictureplasty techniques is determined by several factors, including the quantity of strictures, the length of each stricture, the extent of inflammation in the affected bowel segments, and the interplay between the bowel strictures. Indications for strictureplasty in surgery encompass multiple small bowel strictures, a history of substantial bowel resection exceeding 100 cm, patients suffering from short bowel syndrome, strictures without concurrent inflammatory lesions but accompanied by fistula formation or phlegmon, strictures occurring at previous anastomotic sites, as well as instances involving growth retardation [13, 14]. It is well-established that strictureplasty is contraindicated in patients with sepsis associated with abscess or phlegmon, as well as in cases characterized by severe inflammation leading to diffuse peritonitis. Other contraindications include suspicion of carcinoma, hypoalbuminemia (<2 g/dl), and tension during strictureplasty closure [15]. The Heineke-Mikulicz (HM) strictureplasty represents a traditional approach primarily utilized for addressing short-segment strictures measuring less than 10 cm. Conversely, the Finney strictureplasty is designed for intermediate strictures spanning from 10 to 25 cm in length, employing a side-to-side technique. This procedure involves the creation of a "U"-shaped enterotomy and anastomosis, forming a blind pouch to alleviate the stricture. The Jaboulay strictureplasty, similar to the Finney method, is intended for intermediate bowel strictures. Notably, it differs in terms of the anastomotic site, which involves relatively healthy bowel sections excluding the stricture site. Following the exposure of the antimesenteric border of the bowel, encompassing the stricture site, an enterotomy is performed via a longitudinal incision in a separate healthy bowel segment. The Judd strictureplasty is a valuable technique designed for short-segment strictures accompanied by a fistulous opening. In contrast, the Moskel-Walske-Neumayer strictureplasty is employed to align the constricted distal bowel lumen with the dilated proximal lumen, utilizing a "Y"-shaped enterotomy. The side-to-side isoperistaltic strictureplasty is a procedure intended for lengthy strictures spanning more than 20–25 cm (**Table 2**) [16, 17].

In the past, bypass or exclusion surgery was a common approach for ileocecal Crohn's disease. However, in the current medical landscape, bypass surgery is no longer recommended due to the increased occurrence of septic complications post-surgery and the elevated risk of malignant transformation in the bypassed segment [18].

Endoscopic balloon dilation may be regarded as a viable component within the therapeutic repertoire for addressing obstructive complications of Crohn's disease resulting from strictures. However, it is crucial to exercise caution, as the risk of perforation not only raises morbidity but also elevates the potential for mortality.

2.4 Hemorrhage

Massive intestinal hemorrhage is an uncommon complication associated with terminal ileitis in Crohn's disease. Since the bleeding stems from active disease, individuals with Crohn's disease may experience recurrent episodes, often necessitating surgical intervention. The assessment and management of this complication closely align with approaches used for other causes of gastrointestinal bleeding [19]. In cases where the disease's extent is restricted, as assessed through contrast radiography,

Segment length	Strictureplasty technique
<10 cm	Heineke-Mikulicz strictureplasty
	Judd strictureplasty
	Moskel-Walske-Neumayer strictureplasty
10–25 cm	Finney strictureplasty
	Jaboulay strictureplasty
>25 cm	Side-to-side isoperistaltic strictureplasty
	Michelassi's strictureplasty
	Sasaki strictureplasty

Table 2.
Strictureplasty procedures based on the length of strictures.

deliberation should lean towards elective resection. However, in the presence of persistent and uncontrollable hemorrhaging, it is prudent to pursue an angiogram (typically after a preceding bleeding scan) to precisely identify the bleeding source, especially when multiple disease sites are involved [20].

2.5 Cancer

Individuals afflicted with Crohn's disease face an elevated lifetime risk of developing cancer. The majority of cancers that arise in individuals with Crohn's disease are adenocarcinomas. However, in comparison to de novo cancers, these cancers tend to manifest at a younger age, exhibit a higher prevalence in the distal small bowel, and can often present as multifocal malignancies [21]. The occurrence of cancer is intricately associated with the presence of chronic perineal fistulae and segments of the small bowel that have been excluded from the normal digestive process. Surgeons have traditionally refrained from performing intestinal bypass procedures or leaving excluded intestinal segments in situ for prolonged periods due to the increased susceptibility to cancer development within these bypassed loops, coupled with the inherent difficulties in imaging such segments. Surgical management of small bowel carcinomas in individuals with Crohn's disease primarily involves segmental radical resection, whenever possible. Unfortunately, the prognosis for such cases tends to be grim [22].

2.6 Failure of medical therapy

Approximately one-third of patients undergo surgery for Crohn's disease after failure of medical treatment [4]. In the end, surgical intervention becomes a consideration when all medical avenues have been explored exhaustively. The criteria for medical therapy failure go beyond mere symptom control; it also encompasses cases where patients, even with symptom management, experience intolerable side effects or adverse reactions stemming from their prescribed medications. The timing of intervention plays a pivotal role in averting the worsening of health status, the onset of malnutrition or weight loss, or the requirement for escalating steroid doses, all of which could have substantial adverse effects on surgical results.

2.7 Perforation

Perforation is an exceedingly uncommon event in Crohn's disease. When sepsis, abdominal pain, and diffuse peritonitis are present, emergency surgical intervention is required to manage sepsis effectively. This condition is typically associated with complete obstruction or toxic colitis. Diagnostic laparotomy frequently entails the need for stoma creation following resection. The decision for intestinal resection should be based on surgical findings and the patient's condition [9]. When the perforation is a result of complete obstruction caused by a small bowel stricture, it frequently appears just proximal to the stricture site. In such instances, the optimal therapeutic approach entails resection with primary anastomosis, with potential consideration of a proximal diversion. On the other hand, in cases where the perforation is associated with toxic colitis, it tends to occur at the necrotic segment of the bowel wall. In these scenarios, the advised course of action is total abdominal colectomy with the establishment of an end ileostomy.

2.8 Toxic colitis

Toxic colitis represents a grave and potentially life-threatening condition if not managed appropriately and promptly. Patients with severe colitis typically exhibit signs of systemic toxicity. These individuals present with persistent and frequently bloody diarrhea, as well as abdominal pain that remains unresponsive to medical intervention [23]. With the progression of the condition, toxic colitis can ensue. While this complication is more commonly associated with ulcerative colitis, it's crucial to bear in mind that it can also manifest in individuals with Crohn's disease. Age, gender, and colon perforation are among the factors that affect mortality. In the absence of perforation, the treatment regimen often includes high-dose steroids, bowel rest, and antibiotics. If no improvement is observed, emergency surgery should be promptly carried out. Patients require immediate surgical intervention within a 24–72 hour window. Delaying surgery can have severe repercussions and result in heightened postoperative complications [24]. The preferred surgical procedure for these patients involves performing a total abdominal colectomy with the creation of an end ileostomy.

3. Ulcerative colitis

Ulcerative colitis primarily affects the colon and rectum. While surgical intervention in Crohn's disease is typically palliative, in the case of ulcerative colitis, the complete removal of the colon and rectum offers a curative resolution for the disease. Roughly 25–30% of individuals afflicted with ulcerative colitis (UC) will necessitate surgical intervention during their lifetime [25]. Surgical strategies for UC can be categorized into two main groups: emergency and elective procedures (**Table 3**) [26].

3.1 Toxic megacolon

Toxic megacolon is an infrequent yet potentially fatal condition. The primary contributor to mortality among individuals with ulcerative colitis is toxic megacolon. While toxic megacolon typically arises as a consequence of disease relapse in most patients, it can also manifest as an initial presentation of the condition in some cases. Due to impaired colon motility stemming from the nerve plexus involvement within the muscularis propria layer, colon dilation and subsequent ischemia ensue, leading to the onset of toxic megacolon. It's important to note that colon dilation in isolation does not warrant immediate surgical intervention [26, 27]. "Jalen" criteria in the

Elective	Emergency
Colorectal cancer/dysplasia	Toxic megacolon
Extraintestinal manifestations	Perforation
Intractability to medical treatment	Fulminant colitis
Treatment-related complications	Uncontrolled hemorrhage

Table 3.
Indications for surgery in ulcerative colitis.

clinical diagnosis of toxic megacolon is the most widely used measure. The presence of at least two of these criteria, which include fever >38°C, a heart rate exceeding 120 beats per minute, leukocytosis >10,500/μL, and anemia, in conjunction with at least one of the following: dehydration, electrolyte disturbances, alterations in consciousness, or hypotension, is required. The colon diameter is usually wider than 6 cm. Initially, a regimen of bowel rest, intravenous fluids, broad-spectrum antibiotics, and intravenous steroids should be considered [28]. In the absence of clinical deterioration or significant clinical conditions, the recommended duration for medical treatment is 4–7 days, during which it has been demonstrated that the need for emergency surgery dissipates in 50% of patients [29]. The goal is to eliminate the need for emergency surgery and transition the patient to an elective status. In emergent situations, the primary surgical intervention typically involves a total abdominal colectomy with the creation of an end ileostomy (with or without a mucus fistula). This resection effectively eliminates the majority of the diseased colon [27].

3.2 Perforation

Although the risk of perforation is low in the absence of toxic megacolon, the risk of perforation is high in the first attack. Although rare, its mortality rate is high. The risk of perforation is associated with the severity of the acute attack and the extent of inflammatory conditions within the colon. A direct radiograph usually allows for a diagnosis of free perforation, but in cases of closed perforation, computerized tomography is helpful. Surgical method total colectomy and terminal ileostomy should be preferred [30].

3.3 Fulminant colitis

Fulminant colitis is a condition defined by extensive transmural inflammation of the serosa and systemic manifestations of toxicity. Acute fulminant colitis occurs in approximately 10% of patients with ulcerative colitis [29]. The severity of UC can be classified into categories of mild, moderate, severe, or fulminant, depending on factors such as daily bowel movements, systemic symptoms, and inflammatory markers. It is imperative to routinely evaluate these patients objectively by monitoring parameters like hemoglobin levels, C-reactive protein (CRP) levels, stool frequency, and abdominal imaging. Surgery is typically recommended in cases of clinical deterioration or if significant clinical improvement is not observed within a 7-day timeframe [31]. When a diagnosis of fulminant colitis is established, treatment should be initiated promptly, and if possible, the patient should be monitored under intensive care conditions. In cases of unresponsiveness to medical treatment, emergency colectomy should be performed for the patient [29].

3.4 Uncontrolled hemorrhage

Massive hemorrhage represents another indication for emergency surgery. The bleeding arises from extensive mucosal ulcerations, necessitating abdominal colectomy. For patients who do not respond to resuscitation, the preferred surgical approach is total colectomy, the creation of an end ileostomy, and closure of the rectal stump. Keeping the rectal stump in place preserves the possibility of a future restorative procedure. Nevertheless, it is important to note that bleeding may persist in certain cases where proctectomy was not performed. In such instances, it typically responds to higher doses of systemic steroids, topical steroid administration, or intrarectal tamponade using gauzes soaked in a diluted adrenaline solution. In cases of persistent bleeding, proctectomy should be considered as the recommended course of action [32].

3.5 Colorectal cancer/dysplasia

A diagnosis of dysplasia, dysplasia-associated lesions or invasive carcinoma in a patient with UC is an unequivocal indication for surgery. Patients with ulcerative colitis are recognized to be at a heightened risk of developing colorectal cancer [33]. The likelihood of malignancy rises with extensive colonic involvement and the duration of symptoms, with an estimated risk of approximately 2% at the end of 10 years, 8% at the end of 20 years, and 18% at the end of 30 years [34]. Therefore, the preferred course of action for UC patients presenting with colorectal cancer or high-grade dysplasia is proctocolectomy, either with an end ileostomy or through ileal pouch anal anastomosis. The necessity and timing of surgery in patients with low-grade dysplasia continue to be subjects of intense debate. While low-grade dysplasia has long been considered to carry minimal risk, up to 20% of patients with low-grade dysplasia may have invasive cancer present. Furthermore, patients can advance from low-grade dysplasia to colorectal cancer without any intermediate signs of high-grade dysplasia. It should be noted that when dysplasia of any degree is discovered at colonoscopy, the likelihood of a concomitant carcinoma is high [35]. Nonetheless, it is worth mentioning that a variety of small observational studies have not demonstrated a definitive pattern of dysplasia progression. Consequently, some proponents argue for close endoscopic surveillance as a management strategy for low-grade dysplasia, with surgical intervention reserved for those patients who subsequently develop high-grade dysplasi or colorectal cancer [36, 37]. When low-grade dysplasia is localized to a single lesion, annual colonoscopy suffices. In instances of multifocal occurrence, monitoring every 6 months is recommended, with the patient being educated about the possibility of prophylactic proctocolectomy [34, 38, 39]. In ulcerative colitis, there are two widely accepted elective surgical options: total proctocolectomy with an end ileostomy or restorative proctocolectomy with ileal pouch anal(J,S,W) anastomosis. Various risk factors have been proposed during the postoperative period. In ulcerative colitis, pouch-related septic complications, especially in immunosuppressed patients. Closure of a diverting loop ileostomy is typically carried out 6–8 weeks following confirmation of the intact ileal J-pouch-anal anastomosis. Assessment of the ileal J-pouch is conducted through either a colonoscopy.

3.6 Extraintestinal manifestations

Surgical treatment is seldom required for the extraintestinal symptoms of ulcerative colitis. Among the extraintestinal manifestations that show improvement after colectomy are peripheral arthritis, erythema nodosum, pyoderma gangrenosum, thromboembolic complications, and ocular symptoms like uveitis, iritis, and episcleritis [40].

3.7 Intractability to medical treatment/treatment-related complications

It is the most frequent surgical indication in ulcerative colitis. Prolonging the course of medical treatment in the event of therapeutic failure also diminishes the likelihood of a favorable response to surgical intervention. Patients with chronic, active disease and a short tubular colon due to chronic mucosal inflammation and scarring on radiological assessment should be considered for surgical evaluation and treatment. Patients with ongoing active disease despite a 3-month course of medical treatment or those requiring steroid therapy for more than 12 months should undergo assessment for surgical intervention.

Patients who develop severe side effects or complications during medical treatment are also candidates for surgical intervention. Surgery should be considered for reasons such as bone pathologies, ocular issues, psychiatric problems, and growth retardation that arise due to immunosuppressive therapy [41, 42].

4. Indeterminate colitis

In approximately 5% of cases of inflammatory bowel diseases, a definitive diagnosis of either ulcerative colitis or Crohn's disease cannot be established [43]. The most significant reasons for this are inadequate clinical, radiological, endoscopic, and pathological information or the presence of features showing both ulcerative colitis and Crohn's disease in the patient [44]. In such cases, it is termed indeterminate colitis, which is not a specific disease. Indications for surgery for indeterminate colitis are consistent with ulcerative colitis; It includes incurability, complications from medical treatment, and risk or onset of malignancy. If the diagnosis strongly suggests ulcerative colitis, ileal pouch-anal anastomosis can be performed. In cases where the diagnosis remains unclear, the most logical surgical option is to proceed with completion proctectomy and create an end ileostomy (as in Crohn's colitis) [45].

Author details

Bahadir Kartal
Department of General Surgery, Hitit University, Erol Olcok Training and Research Hospital, Türkiye

*Address all correspondence to: dr.bkartal@hotmail.com

References

[1] Fichera A, Michelassi F. Surgical treatment of Crohn's disease. Journal of Gastrointestinal Surgery. 2007;**11**:791-803

[2] Leowardi C, Heuschen G, Kienle P, et al. Surgical treatment of severe infl ammatory bowel diseases. Digestive Diseases. 2003;**21**(1):54-62

[3] Lynch AC, Delaney CP, Senagore AJ, et al. Clinical outcome and factors predictive of recurrence after enterocutaneous fistula surgery. Annals of Surgery. 2004;**240**:825-831

[4] Hurst RD, Molinari M, Chung TP, et al. Prospective study of the features, indications, and surgical treatment in 513 consecutive patients affected by Crohn's disease. Surgery. 1997;**122**(4):661-667

[5] Alós R, Hinojosa J. Timing of surgery in Crohn's disease: A key issue in the management. World Journal of Gastroenterology. 2008;**14**(36):5532-5539

[6] Berry SM, Fischer JE. Enterocutaneous fistulas. Current Problems in Surgery. 1994;**31**(6):469-566

[7] Tassiopoulos AK, Baum G, Halverson JD. Small bowel fistulas. The Surgical Clinics of North America. 1996;**76**(5):1175-1181

[8] Strong SA. Surgery for Crohn's disease. In: Wolff BG, Fleshman JW, Beck DE, et al., editors. ASCRS Textbook of Colon and Rectal Surgery. New York: Springer; 2007. pp. 584-600

[9] Cellini C, Safar B, Fleshman J. Surgical management of pyogenic complications of Crohn's disease. Inflammatory Bowel Diseases. 2010;**16**:512-517

[10] Gervais DA, Hahn PF, O'Neill MJ, et al. Percutaneous abscess drainage in Crohn disease: Technical success and short- and long-term outcomes during 14 years. Radiology. 2002;**222**(3):645-651

[11] Michelassi F, Balestracci T, Chappell R, et al. Primary and recurrent Crohn's disease. Experience with 1379 patients. Annals of Surgery. 1991;**214**(3):230-238. discussion 238-40

[12] Andrews HA, Keighley MR, Alexander-Williams J, et al. Strategy for management of distal ileal Crohn's disease. British Journal of Surgery. 1991;**78**:679

[13] Van Bodegraven AA, Pena AS. Treatment of extraintestinal manifestations in inflammatory bowel diseases. Current Treatment Options in Gastroenterology. 2003;**6**(3):201-212

[14] Juillerat P, Mottet C, Froehlich F, et al. Extraintestinal manifestations of Crohn's disease. Digestion. 2005;**71**(1):31-36

[15] Ambe R, Campbell L, Cagir B. A comprehensive review of strictureplasty techniques in Crohn's disease: Types, indications, comparisons, and safety. Journal of Gastrointestinal Surgery. 2012;**16**(1):209-217

[16] Campbell L, Ambe R, Weaver J, et al. Comparison of conventional and nonconventional strictureplasties in Crohn's disease: A systematic review and meta-analysis. Diseases of the Colon and Rectum. 2012;**55**(6):714-726

[17] Tichansky D, Cagir B, Yoo E, et al. Strictureplasty for Crohn's disease: Meta-analysis. Diseases of the Colon and Rectum. 2000;**43**:911-919

[18] Alexander-Williams J, Fielding JF, Cooke WT. A comparison of results of excision and bypass for ileal Crohn's disease. Gut. 1972;**13**(12):973-975

[19] Farmer RG. Lower gastrointestinal bleeding in inflammatory bowel disease. Gastroenterologia Japonica. 1991;**26**(Suppl. 3):93-100

[20] Homan WP, Tang CK, Thorbjarnarson B. Acute massive hemorrhage from intestinal Crohn disease. Report of seven cases and review of the literature. Archives of Surgery. 1976;**111**(8):901-905

[21] Frank JD, Shorey BA. Adenocarcinoma of the small bowel as a complication of Crohn's disease. Gut. 1973;**14**(2):120-124

[22] Ribeiro MB, Greenstein AJ, Heimann TM, et al. Adenocarcinoma of the small intestine in Crohn's disease. Surgery, Gynecology & Obstetrics. 1991;**173**(5):343-349

[23] Greenstein AJ, Sachar DB, Gibas A, et al. Outcome of toxic dilatation in ulcerative and Crohn's colitis. Journal of Clinical Gastroenterology. 1985;**7**(2):137-143

[24] Bartels SA, Gardenbroek TJ, Bos L, et al. Prolonged preoperative hospital stay is a risk factor for complications after emergency colectomy for severe colitis. Colorectal Disease. 2013;**15**(11):1392-1398

[25] Andersson P, Soderholm JD. Surgery in ulcerative colitis: Indication and timing. Digestive Diseases. 2009;**27**(3):335-340

[26] Parray FQ, Wani ML, Malik AA, et al. Ulcerative colitis: A challenge to surgeons. International Journal of Preventive Medicine. 2012;**3**(11):749-763

[27] Arnell TD. Surgical management of acute colitis and toxic megacolon. Clinics in Colon and Rectal Surgery. 2004;**17**(1):71-74

[28] Dayan B, Turner D. Role of surgery in severe ulcerative colitis in the era of medical rescue therapy. World Journal of Gastroenterology. 2012;**18**(29):3833-3838

[29] Travis SP, Stange EF, Lémann M, et al. European evidence-based consensus on the management of ulcerative colitis: Current management. Journal of Crohn's & Colitis. 2008;**2**(1):24-62

[30] Hwang JM, Varma MG. Surgery for inflammatory bowel disease. World Journal of Gastroenterology. 2008;**14**(17):2678-2690

[31] Truelove SC, Witts LJ. Cortisone in ulcerative colitis; Final report on a therapeutic trial. British Medical Journal. 1955;**2**(4947):1041-1048

[32] Grucela A, Steinhagen RM. Current surgical management of ulcerative colitis. Mount Sinai Journal of Medicine. 2009;**76**:606-612

[33] Lindberg B, Persson B, Veress B, et al. Twenty years' colonoscopic surveillance of patients with ulcerative colitis. Detection of dysplastic and malignant transformation. Scandinavian Journal of Gastroenterology. 1996;**31**:1195

[34] Eaden JA, Abrams KR, Mayberry JF. The risk of colorectal cancer in ulcerative colitis: A meta-analysis. Gut. 2001;**48**:526-535

[35] Gorfine SR, Bauer JJ, Harris MT, et al. Dysplasia complicating chronic ulcerative colitis: Is immediate colectomy warranted? Diseases of the Colon and Rectum. 2000;**43**:1575

[36] Smith LA, Baraza W, Tiffin N, et al. Endoscopic resection of adenoma-like mass in chronic ulcerative colitis using a combined endoscopic mucosal resection and cap assisted submucosal dissection technique. Inflammatory Bowel Diseases. 2008;**14**(10):1380-1386

[37] Hurlstone DP, Sanders DS, Atkinson R, et al. Endoscopic mucosal resection for flat neoplasia in chronic ulcerative colitis: Can we change the endoscopic management paradigm? Gut. 2007;**56**(6):838-846

[38] Manes G, Imbesi V, Ardizzone S, et al. Appropriateness and diagnostic yield of colonoscopy in the management of patients with ulcerative colitis: A prospective study in an open access endoscopy service. Inflammatory Bowel Diseases. 2008;**14**(8):1133-1138

[39] Sjöqvist U. Dysplasia in ulcerative colitis - Clinical consequences. Langenbeck's Archives of Surgery. 2004;**389**(5):354-360

[40] Langholz E. Current trends in inflammatory bowel disease: The natural history. Therapeutic Advances in Gastroenterology. 2010;**3**(2):77-86

[41] Kuriyama M, Kato J, Fujimoto T, et al. Risk factors and indications for colectomy in ulcerative colitis patients are different according to patient's clinical background. Diseases of the Colon and Rectum. 2006;**49**(9):1307-1315

[42] Hoentjen F, Sakuraba A, Hanauer S. Update on the management of ulcerative colitis. Current Gastroenterology Reports. 2011;**13**(5):475-485

[43] Yantiss RK, Farraye FA, O'Brien MJ, et al. Prognostic significance of superficial fissuring ulceration in patients with severe "indeterminate" colitis. The American Journal of Surgical Pathology. 2006;**30**:165-170

[44] Tanaka M, Riddell R, Saito H, et al. Morphologic criteria applicable to biopsy specimens for effective distinction of inflamatory bowel disease from other forms of colitis and of Crohn's disease from ulcerative colitis. Scandinavian Journal of Gastroenterology. 1999;**34**:55-67

[45] Hurst RD, Gottlieb LJ, Crucitti P, et al. Primary closure of complicated perineal wounds with myocutaneous and fasciocutaneous flaps after proctectomy for Crohn's disease. Surgery. 2001;**130**(4):767-772; discussion 772-3